Resilient
Surviving My Mental Illness
Liz Grace

Sisters Ignited Media and Publishing Inc.

Book Cover by Rachelle Van Ryssen

Published by Sisters Ignited Media and Publishing Inc.

1st edition/ 2023 © Liz Grace

Praise for Resilient

"An inspiring and unforgettable autobiography. The blend of memory-fueled narration and document-supported storytelling gives a rare, real-time peek into the hardest moments of self-harm, loneliness, and thoughts of suicide, resulting in an important portrait of intense experience that will resonate with readers who have either struggled with mental illness, or have had their life touched by it. This is a remarkably honest, fearless, and selfless piece of writing, one that could help people facing a myriad of challenges, which could even be life-saving." – *Self-Publishing Review,* ★★★★½

"Liz Grace's unflinching account sheds much-needed light on these struggles, making Resilient an incredibly valuable read for anyone who knows someone battling mental illness." - *Books That Make You*

"Grace's transformation from someone battling the shadows of her mind to thrive is a testament to the possibility of recovery and growth." - *Books That Make*

You

"An honest and inspiring account of a young woman's struggles with deafness and mental illness." - *Kirkus Reviews*

"Best book I have read in a while." – Kimberley Muka Powers, author of *A Mind Restored*

"This book will be life changing for many." – *Rachelle van Ryssen, Author, CEO Sisters Ignited Media and Publishing*

"This compelling book is hard to put down." – *Helen diFolco, Occupational Therapist*

"I'm gob smacked at all that you have endured over the years. Your hearing loss and the work it took to adjust to the cochlear implants and learn to interpret all the sounds... felt huge to me. But toss in the mental health challenges, treatment at hospitals, attempts to find a medication mixture that would manage symptoms, be in and out of hospital and still go to school and work ... it's truly mind boggling." – *Cathy Rusling, Occupational Therapist*

"This book will make you uncomfortable, but that's a good thing. Liz takes us on a mental illness journey that most people would find unbearable. The book begins with lots of journal entries that give us insight into how Liz goes through her daily life. The imagery and emotions are overwhelming, but that's the point. I almost put the book away because I found the journal entries difficult to read. They were heavy, confrontational, and depressing. But they prepared me for the rest of the book, so I'm glad I stuck with it.

Any one who's ever had a mental illness or had/has loved ones with a mental illness should read this book. It will help give readers a perspective on what people with schizoaffective disorder go through. Bravo to Liz for sharing her story." – *Steven Shelton, The Mangled Mind Podcast*

"Liz Grace gives the reader a front row seat into her truths as she shares her experiences with mental illness with the added hampering of hearing loss. Her easy-to-read writing style artfully includes some of her own in-the-moment journal entries. Both of which kept me turning the pages. Liz gives the reader – parent, family friend, stranger or professional – valuable insights that could help all involved better understand how to help a person go form "suffering" to "surviving" and even "thriving" with a mental illness, let alone her helpful and fascinating insight into the world of hearing loss. I'm glad I braved reading about Liz's experiences. She's making others more aware of how we can do better and help others." – *Kathleen Kline, Editor, Author, Owner of Dragonfly Editing and Publishing*

"I found her experience with implants to be fascinating, enlightening, and much different than I expected."
– *Bethany Yeiser, author of Mind Estranged and President of CURESZ Foundation*

Author Bio

LIZ GRACE IS A first-time author in recovery from Schizoaffective Disorder who lives with the daily challenges of profound hearing loss. Starting at the age of sixteen, she gradually lost her hearing, learned American Sign Language in university and at age twenty-six, was implanted with bilateral cochlear implants.

Dedication

*A special thanks to all of the people who have contributed and
supported my resilience:
To my grandparents, who showed me the meaning of
unconditional love.
My family, who never gave up on me.
My friends and supports, who were there when
I needed them.*

*To all the support-people of those with illnesses,
may you remember that every action makes a difference,
no matter how big or small.*

To all the people battling illnesses, may you carry on.

Contents

Introduction

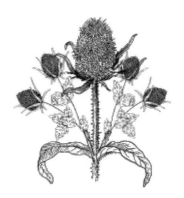

When I developed crippling anxiety after starting a new job, I knew I needed to do something about it and began to see a therapist. As we started to work together, the stress caused me to become hypomanic, and I began writing. This book began as therapeutic writing for myself as I worked through the trauma from my mental illness. As my writing progressed, I joked about the possibility of me writing a book… and then the possibility became a reality—a book began to evolve. From the first 23,000 words I wrote in twenty-four hours while manic, to the umpteenth edit before the final submission,

I poured my heart, my soul, and my life experiences into this book.

To ensure that the content of the book was accurate, I requested and received all of my chart notes from every hospitalization over the past eighteen years. This came at a costly price both emotionally (due to re-reading through the notes) and financially (as obtaining these records came with a hefty fee). It was bittersweet reading through the notes. The bitter being re-experiencing my own inner distress and the hurdles with being mistreated by some of the professionals/staff who I encountered. The sweet, being reminded of the family, friends and professionals who helped to rebuild and piece me back together.

This is a book for families and workers who are trying to understand mental illness. It is for people living with mental illness; to know you are not alone. As a story of hope and resilience despite dark times, this book emphasizes the importance of valuing people who want to help. This isn't always easy or comfortable to read, just as it isn't easy or comfortable to live.

I wrote this book to help the reader step into my shoes to understand my experience, and I want the reader to truly understand what was going through my mind, my thoughts, my feelings, and my insecurities. There are times you may feel confused, and it may seem as if information is missing. This memoir reflects my lived experience, where all too often my life felt like it was missing pieces. Please practice self-care while reading this book.

I pieced this story together from my own memories and journals, what I have been told by others, and the information I could access in my health records. I have changed and/or outright removed some names and places to protect the privacy of others. It is important to note that my memories of these experiences may differ from the memories of others.

When reading, please note that all journal quotes are *italicized.*

<u>Content warning</u> - This story describes experiences of suicide, suicidal ideation, self-harm, and restraints.

Prologue

March 2022

Today I am feeling energetic—abnormally so. At thirty-four years of age, my thoughts are moving fast and I'm literally bouncing around. Usually, my alarm wakes me at 5:45 a.m., but today I'm up at 5. By 5:30 a.m., I'm showered and drinking tea in front of the fireplace. At 7:15 a.m., I pack my lunch and load the car. At 7:30 a.m. I'm on the road. I get velocitized when my mood is up like this, as a result I'm careful to check my speed often. When there's another car on the road, I keep pace with it to keep my speed steady. I use cruise control when it's safe to do so.

All my senses are on high alert. The sun is only just coming up, but I'm wearing sunglasses. The music in the car is loud enough for me to feel it: when I get to town, I will lower it. Any tightness in my pants will bother me throughout the day, so I'm wearing a size too big.

I arrive at work at 7:52. By 7:55 a.m. I'm in my office and clocked in. I jump into working right away, signing into the Electronic Medical Record, followed by checking my email. I finish some notes and prepare for my first client at nine.

Closer to 8:30 a.m., as people come in, they will say hi as they walk past. I'm Deaf, but I usually hear most of them with the help of my cochlear implants, and I greet them in return. At 8:45 a.m., I prepare for my first client of the day, an initial occupational therapy assessment for a lady with fibromyalgia. When my schedule shows that she has arrived on time, just before 9 a.m., I'm ready to get into OT mode. I close my eyes and take a few deep breaths. My brain is still on high speed, but it's time to slow my mind; slow my body. My racing heart calms a little, and at 9 a.m. I escort her from the waiting room back to my office. I make a conscious effort to slow my speech and not rush. I assess her gait and mobility as we walk slowly down the hall. I focus on letting her do the talking. I encourage her to tell me her story, what's bothering her, and what she would like to change. Patient input and involvement is key to a positive outcome—this I know as both a professional and a patient. I guide our discussion, and by 9:30 a.m., we're formulating her goals. We book our next appointment in two weeks, and I walk her out at 9:50 a.m. She leaves with a plan, and I hope, the beginning of a successful strategy.

I know things are starting to move faster and faster in my mind. I want to—need to—keep in control of it this time.

Part One

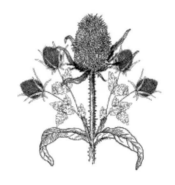

Chapter 1

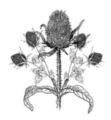

S UMMER 2005

As I walk in the door, returning home from camp, I notice them sitting at the kitchen table, hand-in-hand.

"We're getting married!"

Just like that, I find out simultaneously that not only are they dating, but they have been dating long enough to be getting married. He didn't bother to tell me. I'm seventeen, I am trying to catch my breath as the surge of my emotions literally knocks the wind out of me.

The announcement of my father's plan to marry comes as a total shock to me. I feel betrayed that he didn't think it was important enough to tell me they had been dating. For the past seven years, I have simply moved on, never having been taught how to grieve my mother's death. Through no fault of my own, or really anyone's at all, the adults in my life failed to teach me the necessary emotional functions required to grieve and respond to the death of my mother in a healthy manner.

I'm not sure what reaction my father and his fiancé Janet are expecting me to give? An open arms welcome to a woman I know nothing about, other than her name, while dealing with the loss of my mother? I am distressed.

I go upstairs to my room following this announcement in a mix of shock and sadness while attempting to keep it together. I am suddenly faced with the fact that my mother is actually gone, even if this is just a subconscious thought. As a response to this unsettling news, I do the one thing I know will help to release some of my pain. I take a razor and push the sharp blade deep into the skin on my upper arm. I feel the sharp cut; I observe the red blood emerge and spill. I know I need to escape my home and race off to James' house (a guy from cadets who I am currently dating).

"Please don't cut yourself again," he pleads as he holds me in his arms.

I wish it were that easy.

"What do you know about her?" my boyfriend asks.

"Around 2004–2005", I explain, "I noticed my dad was gone more often. Normally he'd be home, working on the computer, but lately he had been out of the house. After a few months, he told me he was giving someone computer lessons and, as far as I knew, that was all they were; teacher and student."

I continue my story, "Janet began to show up around the house more and more often. I knew little about her except she had three kids, who our family used to swim with, and she knew my mother."

I explain that at one point, my older sister Jennifer, who was away at university, asked me, "Is Dad dating?"

"I don't think so," I had told her. "He told us he was giving someone computer lessons but hasn't said anything else." I wrap up my story.

"I guess he thought I could mind read as he never bothered to tell me he was dating." I clarify, "If he had communicated this to me, I would have been happy for him as I always anticipated he would remarry."

I tell James, "It is the lack of respect with him not telling me that was so hurtful."

When my sister moved away to school in 2002, I got to have her bedroom. This was two years ago when, for the first time, I had privacy. I was fifteen years old then. After sharing a bedroom for years with a sibling, I craved my own space and finally had it.

Now I am seventeen, I live at home with my dad, my younger sister Danielle, and my older brother Brian. My mother had been thirty-seven years young, lively, and a mother to four children. She died of breast cancer just before I turned ten years old. After her death, I was raised by my father, my maternal grandparents, and, quite frankly, I raised myself.

My father's impending marriage forces me, for the first time in seven years, to come face to face with my mother's death and attempt to grieve it. I fall even further into a dark hole of despair—depression within me magnified.

I do not have the skills to deal with the emotions I am suddenly experiencing. I'll explain it a different way. If you give a seventeen-year-old a calculus problem but that seventeen-year-old only has the math education of a ten-year-old, how do you expect them to solve it? They will try to solve it with the ten-year-old's math mindset, if they even attempt to try to solve it. They don't even have a concept of calculus. Consequently, it's unrealistic to expect them to use calculus skills. This is basically where my emotional development is during this time; I don't have a concept of how to handle my complex emotions, for this reason I use what I know.

Unfortunately, I subconsciously cut Janet out of my life, reacting to the whole situation with the emotional mentality of a ten-year-old. When she enters the room; I leave. I don't look at her. I don't talk to her. I no longer care, and I begin to cut daily. There are many reasons for cutting. Sometimes I feel I am bad and need to be punished, especially if I make a mistake. No one else is giving me any discipline (or praise, for that matter). I can do what I want, and no one seems to care if I come home at eleven p.m. on a school night. So, I start to punish myself. Other times I cut because I need to release the pent-up pain. I haven't cried a real cry since my mom's death, and I don't know how. I have emotions in my body that are causing depression, anxiety, and I need them out. Thus, cutting is the only way which helps me to release these pent-up emotions.

Currently when at school, I spend all of class scribbling in my journal, writing "I hate myself" and "I am bad."

One teacher takes note of this and takes the time after class one day to find out what is bothering me. I explain to her my dad is getting remarried. I begin to cry but then quickly shut down, as I refuse to let anyone see what I am feeling. I wear long sleeves in the summer, claiming I'm always cold (which I am), but in reality, I wear the long sleeves to hide the cuts. Unfortunately, either no one realizes that my mental health is so bad or they realize and don't know how to help me. Or, worse, they just don't care. So, I continue on without adult support.

My friends are great and very supportive. I am a part of the local cadet squadron, which is basically a youth group led by military personnel. Very much like a military boy-scouts but without the badges and add in some ranks. The squadron has a Commanding Officer who is a Major in the air force and several lower-ranking air force and civilian adults who help run the program. The cadets are youth between the ages of twelve to eighteen and have their own ranking system with levels of responsibility. I am involved with training the new recruits. I teach classes on various subjects (military ranks, basic aviation, drill), and while I never have the interest to pursue it, there is the option to take 'ground school' (where you learn about flying) and obtain a glider or pilot's licence for free.

My friends and the routine keep me sane during this time, more so than anyone, except for maybe my grandparents, who will become a huge part of my life. My friends talk to me, listen to me, and get me out of my house, where I am not doing well. Cadets is something

I excel at. It's several evenings a week and involves rules and discipline. It gives me leadership opportunities and enables me to develop my natural leadership skills.

My family isn't so supportive. My brother in particular is determined that I'm a loser and he thinks the cadets is stupid. He never misses an opportunity to tell me that something is 'dumb' or 'stupid,' and he will continue to do this well into adulthood.

• • ● ●• ● ● • •

Early 1990s

I come from a family with four children. My older sister Jennifer is four years older than me; my brother Brian is two years older than me, and my younger sister Danielle is four-and-a-half years younger. I was born in 1987, making me a Millennial, and we lived in a town called Pickering, which bordered Toronto to the west and Lake Ontario at the south end. There were a lot of wetlands nearby, including a large bay called Frenchman's Bay, and we were just a few kilometres from the GO train station, which was the commuter train into downtown Toronto. Pickering had a nuclear power plant in operation while I was growing up. When we were kids, we used to have emergency preparedness drills at school to practice evacuating and handing out iodine pills. My brother and I used to joke that we were in the 'instant death zone,' meaning if there ever was to be an accident, we were so close we would be instantly killed. I don't know if this was true or not, but joking about it was our way of dealing with it.

My family had a happy relationship when I was young, and my young self was not aware of any conflicts in the home. Though there was plenty of sibling rivalry, and I struggled with sharing a room.

• • • ● ● • ● ● • •

Summer 2005

While I am away at an overnight cadet camp in the summer, just before my dad's marriage announcement, a staff member recognizes the signs of my poor mental health. I speak with a counsellor at the camp briefly and she recommends some counselling when I get home. She helps me find a local counsellor who works with youth. I don't have to pay anything for the service for a limited number of sessions.

My journaling becomes more regular, and my entries become quite disturbing and rather jumbled, my thoughts not always making sense.

At first, I am afraid of meeting with a counsellor. I know it will be a social worker and I don't want to be put on drugs. I am already suicidal, wishing I could slit my wrists, but I'm afraid of my legacy being that I committed suicide. I can't have that.

Journal Entry: Thursday, September 8th, 2005

Today will be my first appointment with (I thought) the counsellor. It turns out it is actually a group intake. I'm worried. Will they think I'm crazy and want to lock me up? What if they want to put me on drugs or something crazy like that? Some days, I want to take the blade and just slit my wrists, but I don't want to get that title. I want to die because of something that wasn't my fault. Like a drunk driver. That would be perfect.

At the intake, the social workers give us (a small group of teenagers) a few questionnaires to fill out. I'm bouncing my legs from my anxiety, and I fill the questionnaires out truthfully. Yes, I am hurting myself. Yes, my mood is poor. Yes, I have anxiety. The social workers finish by talking to each of us one-on-one to get an idea of what program would benefit us. I am left for last, and they spend longer with me than the other teens. They want to know about the cutting. They ask if I am suicidal; they ask if I am safe. I must satisfy the requirements to not be 'incurable,' as I am signed up for some programs (individual counselling and a group program).

I also begin to think I am fat and don't deserve to take up space in this world. I can't stand eating but I feel sick when I don't. I'm feeling hopeless about my future; I know I have to go to university because it is expected of me. But I don't want to, I feel that I will never accomplish anything. The world would be better off if I just didn't exist.

Journal Entry: Monday, September 12th, 2005

You are going to be fat and gross and even more disgusting. I hate my life. I feel gross when I don't eat and even grosser when I do eat. Why do I even bother to try to do schoolwork? I'm not going to university. You've known it from the start. You just picked something so that no one would question you about why you haven't picked something or 'don't you want to go to university' and stuff like that. And you can't say "No" to that. It's not socially appropriate. If you don't go to university and get a job and have a family, you are a terrible mom for your family. A disappointment. Failure. You are forgotten about. Never mentioned again. Nobody knows you, nobody likes you. Nobody could care if you are dead. I want to die before they find out that I won't succeed. I don't know if I don't want to succeed. I just know that I won't. I can't. It's impossible with my "study habits". Sometimes I'll try to change them, but most of the time I just don't care. I don't really know what I'll be doing in 3 years. I don't even know what I'll be doing next year. Sure, I know what I'll be "doing". In Uni. But that is what I tell people. Not what I truly believe. I think I'd rather not exist. But I want to see what's going on. I just don't want to exist. I wonder if I ran away, telling people I was going to Uni, then I could be gone forever. No one would know me, no one would see me. But eventually, when the bills go unpaid or something, someone would notice me. I just need to sleep and have all of this crap stop.

Within a few days, my anxiety and depression worsen. Life is feeling more and more unfair. I don't realize I'm doing things wrong, but apparently, I am. This gets me, for the first time in seven years, punishment. Punishment for things I have always done. Punishment for things I don't know are wrong. Punishment that seems unfair for what I have done. Since I am a perfectionist, I feel I must punish myself for needing to be punished. I wish they would just tell me the problem; I would change it if I knew! My friends are what's keeping me together. When my father takes away my internet cable (which to me is an extreme punishment for leaving some books on the table), I am incredibly isolated. I have no coping mechanism other than to cut, so this is what I do.

I don't know why, but today was a bad day for me. First, I was freaking out during bio when that lady sat beside me. The student teacher. I dunno. And then I got home and, of course, didn't do any homework. Instead, I ate 2 pizza pops and told myself I'd clean my room. Did I? Of course not! And when I went out later to get vitamins, I came back to chaos. I got in trouble as soon as I walked in the door for having my stuff on the table. My dad took away my internet cable. I'm not sure how this is a fair punishment for leaving books on the table when I have never been told not to and everyone in the house does it. I had left my journal in my bag, and now I know my dad has been in my room *shudders*. I was so upset after all that I cut, and it took me about an hour to get everything to stop bleeding. I hated not having my internet. I was sooo isolated! I never want that to happen again.

With every cut that I make, the cuts get deeper. I feel more and more need to make myself hurt; to make myself bleed. I deserve it.

Journal Entry: Tuesday, September 13th, 2005

I had a really bad night last night. I went to the store for vitamins and deodorant. When I got home, my dad was cleaning off the table and was mad at me. I went upstairs, and he had taken the internet cord, so I was really really panicking, so I cut. I cut badly. I think I cut a vein. It took an hour to stop bleeding and then it really really hurt more than normal. It made my hand tingle, and there were parts of the cut that I couldn't feel.

I went to bed exhausted and a little dizzy. I woke up at 5:00 a.m. and it was bleeding again, so now I have to clean my room and wash my sheets. I was supposed to clean yesterday, but I didn't and I'm really upset that I let myself eat all that crap and I didn't even clean. Bad Bad Bad. No wonder you are so fat this morning. Bad Bad Bad. You deserve that cut. Yuck. This morning was bad too. You took too long to get up and then your cut hurt in the shower.

In my first true counselling session just a few days after the intake, I meet the social worker who I will be working with. Her name is Evalyn. I worry about opening up; what if I start to talk about things but we just leave them alone? How will I deal with this can that is now open?

Journal Entry: Wednesday, September 14th, 2005

Today I attended an individual counselling session with a Social Worker named Evalyn. I worry about talking about so many sensitive topics and then never dealing with them. I feel it is easier to leave them shut, and this makes it hard for me to open up. This does, however, help me see how depressed and anxious I really am.

I have a job as 'third staff' at a group home for medically complex children. My role is more of the housekeeping and changing diapers for the younger children. I enjoy, as much as I can enjoy my job in my current mental state, the work as it relates to the medical field. I bike to school in the morning, about eight kilometres away. In the afternoon I bike to work, then home after that. Some evenings I go for an overnight shift, where I sleep in the basement until the morning.

Journal Entry: Thursday, September 15th, 2005

Today I am struggling. I find it hard getting up, hard to bike to school and don't want to work at the children's group home where I recently started. I have also started to get dizzy, probably because I am barely eating.

I hate life so much that I just want to no longer exist. I am struggling to bike to school and to work. My motivation is in the pits. And, because I don't eat, I keep getting dizzy.

I hate my life. I just want to curl up in my bed and die. I want my life to be non-existent. I just want it to not be there (sic). I don't want to be. I want to curl up in bed and be gone. I can't deal with my stupid life. I miss being at camp. I could forget about my home problems there.

My thoughts move toward the idea of suicide, but I don't want the negative stigma that is associated with having killed myself.

I don't want to exist here. Suicide is such a dirty word. It's more like de-existing yourself. You die internally, so you put the body to rest, and make it die too. Die. I don't like that word either. Reminds me too much of … other stuff (sic). I want to go away and never come back. I want to be unknown, so I can de-exist myself with no one knowing. But that's impossible. There will always be someone who knows your name, even if they don't care. So long as your name exists, you exist. You can't de-exist yourself, only to have your name exist, with a curse on it. The curse of the label "Suicide".

When it comes to my mood, I find I barely enjoy anything anymore and feel hopeless and unmotivated. My attention is poor.

I can barely sit down and do cadet stuff, and I at least kind of enjoy that. But school work? I just don't know. Or even really care. Really, I just don't care. I'm not going to university. I will accomplish nothing with my 'life'. I don't want to exist. I don't want to be here. I don't want to go to work tonight. I want to go to my room. But I don't want to be disturbed. I just want to be alone, which makes no sense because I hate being alone. Because I hate being alone. I cut if/when I feel alone. Nothing makes sense. Nothing makes sense. Maybe I'm going crazy.

My mood is getting worse and worse.

Journal Entry: Friday, September 16th, 2005

I want to curl up into a ball and cry. But I can't. I can't cry. I'm screaming inside my head, inside my mind, and I can't do anything about it. Nobody cares. I deserve to rot alone in my stupid life. I don't deserve to be among the living. I'm dead inside. I am nothing. Nothing nothing nothing. I shouldn't be writing this. It's stupid. These are my problems. I need to learn to deal with them myself. Not throw them at other people. I'm stupid.

My mood goes up and down, or rather, neutral and down. I don't really feel happy anymore. But today is the weekend, so I don't have to think about school.

Journal Entry: Saturday, September 17th, 2005

Today I'm only 'not-sad'. Not happy. Just 'not-sad'.

I'm getting more in control of the cutting. I'm trying so hard to stop and no longer do it where other people are around. But the blades still give me comfort over my anxiety. Knowing I could cut if I wanted. I'm still, in the back of my mind, thinking about killing myself as a way to get out of this. I'm getting more of an understanding of my brain. I have recognized that nothing feels good like it used to, even cadets. I'm used to ups and downs, but now I feel the downs more than the ups.

Journal Entry: Sunday, September 18th, 2005

Today I noticed that work is good for me. Two weeks ago I would have freaked out if I felt like cutting but was somewhere where I couldn't do it. I am trying so hard to stop and now, I'm kinda relieved, because I know I won't do it at work. I do not cut in front of others, only when I am feeling alone, or feel like I need to be punished, and sometimes if I just need to feel something other than bad or nothing at all.

Every time I consider not carrying my blades around with me, I imagine myself having another panic attack and then killing myself. It kind of scares me that I brought home an entire bottle of Tylenol. I'm not sure why. I have Tylenol at home, even if it's not the easy tabs. I think in the back of my mind it was in case I decide to kill myself. And that scares me too. But ya, this afternoon, when I was walking, I had these "revelations". First, I really don't enjoy anything as much. I consider everything about 3 steps lower than what it should be. Work is 'ok'; Cadets I 'like', not love; school I 'loathe with a passion', and home I 'hate'. I guess I'm just 'depressed' and 'anxious'.

Previously I would have a really high point, followed by a low point. But lately the highs aren't as high, and the lows are much lower than before. Eventually they have stopped becoming high at all, just the least-low part of the day/week/month.

In school, I sit in the back row in English class. This suits me, as I am anxious about having someone behind me. However, the teacher now wants to change our seating plan. My anxiety skyrockets and I can no longer think straight. I no longer feel in control.

Journal Entry: Monday September 19th, 2005

In English we changed spots. I'm no longer at the back. I can't concentrate. I freaked out in my head so much! Then, of course, I have to work tonight so I can't unwind before work. I feel like I want to quit, but I don't know if that's me or the 'depression/anxiety' talking. How can I feel these things but I can't control them?

The next day becomes my newest low. I begin to think, very superficially, about killing myself. I don't have any intention to do it right now, but the thought occurs to me, and I wonder if that might be the ultimate solution to my problems.

Journal Entry: Tuesday, September 20th, 2005

Today my mood dropped further, and it's weird. I just walked from school to the bus stop, and all I can think about is killing myself. Not 'not existing' but actual suicide. I think I have a plan, but at this time I don't have any plans to follow through with it. I'll gather my medications in case I do; bottles of Tylenol, expired medications, Gravol, to prevent throwing up. If those don't work, I will slit my wrists.

Chapter 2

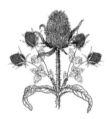

WEDNESDAY, SEPTEMBER 21ST, 2005

"I have the pills should I choose to take them,"
I say to Evalyn during my session with her.

I am unaware that this is automatically going to require her to force me to go to the hospital. We talk
about my plan some more, not realizing that with this
conversation, I am digging myself into a deeper hole. She
gets another social worker and together they ask me the
same questions.

"So, you've been collecting some pills? Why don't you
tell me about them?" the other social worker asks.

"I have collected some Tylenol, some expired medications, some Gravol…" I nonchalantly repeat.

"Where did you get the expired meds?" the social
worker asks.

"I picked them up from a table in school. They were just left there," I share.

"And you plan to do this ... when... where?" she asks.

"I don't plan to do it yet," I insist.

"We're going to take you to the ER anyway." Evalyn instructs me. "You really must go to the ER,"

I begin to hyperventilate and shake and feel like my world is closing in on me. We are sitting in Evalyn's office, but I get up to leave. They direct me into the group room.

"I cannot go to the hospital," I say. I feel like curling up under the table, but settle for looking out the window instead.

"Liz, you have a choice right now. You can go in an ambulance..."

"NO WAY!" I scream silently.

"... or you are going in my car," Evalyn states kindly.

"You can just let me go home. I really do need to go to cadets tonight." I offer as an alternative.

"No. If you leave now, I have to call the police. And if you don't go to the ER with me, now, in my car, I will have to call the police to help me get you to the ER."

"I really don't need to... I really just need to go home so I can go to cadets tonight. I'm not planning on doing anything else."

I try, but I cannot convince her to let me leave without her calling the cops, consequently I give in and go with her in her car to the hospital, which is not far away. I am sure that I can convince them I don't need to be admitted. My heart is pounding, and I am on high alert. My worst fear is happening. What if they lock me up and never let me out? What if they force medications on me? I cannot stay in the hospital. Anxiety builds further.

At the ER, they bring us to a small room off the waiting room with a large window facing the hall. There is a small leather loveseat and some hard chairs. Evalyn sits on a chair, and I sit on the love seat. My anxiety is in overdrive. I am shaking and my mind is going a million miles an hour. We seem to wait forever, and eventually, first a triage nurse, then a crisis nurse comes to talk to me. Evalyn does all the talking, explaining what I said, how I have a plan, and how she is concerned for my safety. I'm in a panic. My legs are shaking non-stop.

The doctor comes in and Evalyn repeats the same story. My anxiety is continuously getting higher, and Evalyn only has to talk for a couple of minutes before the doctor decides to admit me. I panic. I need to get out of that room. I try to leave, but get forced into the chair by a security guard and a paramedic. As soon as they are far enough away, I bolt again. I almost make it to the sliding door in the ambulance bay when they grab me. I am forced back into the room. The doctor is there and then the nurse from triage is there, then when I try to bolt again, they pick me up, put me on the couch, and sit on me. Two large men sitting on me, I'm completely unable to move while having a panic attack. They try to restrain me with their weight and give me medicine.

Needles. They want to give me a needle. I think.

"No, no… no," I say as the nurse comes near. "Get off of me!"

"The only way these men will get off of you is if you promise to calm down and not run," the doctor says.

"Okay... okay... but no needles! No needles! I don't want any needles."

I swallow my anxiety and force myself to stay there. I will not have a needle.

My anxiety is on hyperdrive. I am physically being forced to stay here.

Not wanting to be held down, I agree.

"Here, take this. It will help you calm down."

A nurse tries to give me a pill to calm down. I shake my head and tighten my lips. Again, I am not willing to take it because of an overwhelming fear of being medicated and locked up.

"Get a stretcher with restraints, place it outside the door," the doctor orders.

I can see it through the door and the window, lingering there, a constant threat if I cannot control myself. The bed is just a stretcher, the kind you would find in an ER, but it has four baby blue cuffs: two for the wrists and two for the ankles. The thought of being strapped down causes my heart to race and my breath to catch once again. By this point, however, I have figured out that if I swallow my anxiety, deny it, and cover it up; they will not force these barbaric devices on me.

In my mind, I am panicking. *They want to give me needles to calm me. I can't do that. No needles. No, no, no.* I think to myself. They want to give me a pill to make me a little calmer, but I say no. *They want me to be calm. Okay. I can do that. I know how to calm myself.* I try to pull out my blades out of my jacket pocket, to cut, as this is the only way I know how to calm down.

"Give me the razors," the nurse demands. I clench my fist, pulling my hand to my torso. "If you don't give those up, Liz, these men will have to put you in restraints," she threatens.

"But I could use them to calm myself down!"

"No, no, no, no, we can't let you do that, Liz. We won't let you do that."

"Do you have any more of these on you?" the nurse asks.

They try to give me a pill, again, but I won't take it, for what if they are actually trying to poison me? I can't trust them.

I know it is a Wednesday, cadet night, therefore I have to call and let them know I will not be coming. The nurse allows me to use the phone in the hallway. I say nothing about the hospital. The hospital calls my father, who comes to the waiting room, and it seems my brother picks up the car from the counsellor's office. My father says nothing when he comes to the hospital room I am now in. He just sits in the room with me. I guess unsure of what to do or say, barely making eye contact. He sits with me until I am transferred.

The ambulance ride to the other hospital is quiet, mostly. It is just the nurse and me. I sit in a seat, not on the stretcher.

"I used to work on the unit that you will be staying in. It is nice. They will help you," she assures me.

My anxiety is still in overdrive. I want out. I need out. I cannot go into the hospital. When we arrive, I nearly bolt again as I'm getting out of the ambulance. An image of the stretcher with restraints flashes before my eyes, and I don't bolt. My father followed the ambulance in his van. There are also security guards from the hospital that have met us at the ambulance bay, and I don't think I am fast enough in my current state to outrun them. I can drag my feet, though. I'm escorted to a back elevator and to up to the tenth floor, where there is a specialized children's mental health unit.

"Go on" my dad encourages me to walk into the unit when I hesitate. It is the first words he has said to me all night.

I do not want to go in and try desperately to figure out how I can escape.

In the unit, I am met by a nurse named Sherry. She has a no-nonsense attitude and speaks to me as though I am in trouble.

"Dad," she turns to my father, "I'm just going to get her settled in. It's late. You can go now." She turns to me, "Here, put this on," she orders.

It is 10:30 at night and she takes all of my belongings. I am given a gown and permitted to keep my socks and underwear, but they take away my under-wire bra.

"I'm going to lock all of your belongings into this cupboard" she is matter of fact in her tone as she closes and locks the cupboard in my room. "Before I go, I want you to take this." I am once again offered a pill.

"No" I shake my head, refusing to speak.

"It's just a sleeping pill. It will help you relax and sleep," she informs me. I shake my head. "Then go lay down and go to sleep."

There, in this small room, is a single bed that is bolted to the floor. I am scared. Scared of so many things. My mind is flipping through every negative possibility that could arise from the situation, and I wonder why I didn't just keep my mouth shut.

I refuse to go to bed, even though it is late, and sit on the window ledge. The ledge is just long enough for me to sit on and about a foot wide. The glass is so thick there is no possibility that I could punch through it with my bare hands or feet, so there is no safety risk.

"Are you sure you don't want something to help you sleep?" the nurse offers again.

I shake my head. I refuse, as I still do not trust them.

"Okay. It's lights out time. You should lay down and get some rest now. I'm sure it's been a long day. Come on, get in bed at the very least."

They get me to go to bed, but I do not sleep at all.

Thursday, September 22nd, 2005

I barely sleep all night, and I wake up early the next morning. I am forced to get up and go to the dining room. I am now pissed about being here and refuse to cooperate. I refuse to talk to anyone or eat anything. This is partially out of control and partially as I am worried about gaining weight, even though I am 5'7" and 123 lbs. I'm given a menu to fill out for food for the next day, but I refuse to do so as I will not be here that long.

I am very stressed about being locked away, and as such I pace the unit for hours. It is only a small unit, six private bedrooms with bathrooms, a nursing station, a TV room, dining/activity room, and a schoolroom. I am constantly pacing round and round the hallway. Every time I walk by the door, I look out the tiny window, wondering how I can escape.

"I am tired of seeing you up there near those doors. If you don't stop walking up there by the doors, I'm going to put you in restraints," one of the other staff members says.

Another threat of physical restraint.

Just like my room, each room has a window with a window ledge big enough to sit on about three feet off the ground and inside the solid glass of the window. The bedrooms all have a window that faces the hall, and each window has blinds that staff can open from the hallway. This is how the staff check on patients at night when we are supposed to be sleeping. The staffing usually consists of one or two nurses and one or two child and youth workers. During the day, a psychiatrist, a social worker, and a teacher also come on the unit for brief periods of time.

All patients must wear hospital gowns and pants. It is freezing in the unit, but the staff don't care. The adult unit next door has dressing gowns with long sleeves, but the staff refuse to let me have one. So, I freeze. I try to bring a blanket out of my bedroom, but they don't let me. I have goosebumps going up my arms. I don't understand why they won't let be warm. Maybe it is a form of control? Maybe they think I can hide something under the blanket? Regardless, I am forced to stay out of my bedroom, freezing, and getting more and more worked up with every minute.

While not eating my breakfast, I palm a plastic knife, which I hide in my room. My only coping skill is to cut. I know nothing else. I do not steal the knife because I am defiant or want to hurt anyone. It is a survival mechanism for me; the only way I know how to cope with the stress and anxiety is to cut. And while a plastic knife will not cut me, the scratching will provide at least a little relief.

I go into the bathroom, shut the door, and scratch myself to relieve some of my distress. A nurse checks on me and catches me. She takes away the knife and I may no longer close the bathroom door, which faces the door and window to my room. As a result, I now have zero privacy to even go to the bathroom.

My distress is not relieved and accelerates. I seek another way to hurt myself to relieve the emotional pain and anxiety. Now, I notice they have attached baby blue restraints to my bed, like a threat. I am scared of them despite their pale blue colour but also desperate to relieve my distress, and I notice there is a pin on a belt-buckle type mechanism. I try to use it to scratch my skin, but am quickly caught and threatened to be put in restraints if I don't stop. I'm not offered any alternative but to stew in my own anxiety and distress. At some point, someone offers me an elastic to snap against my wrist, as though that is supposed to provide any comparable relief.

Later in the day, a nurse tries to talk to me, and I relent and talk to her a bit. She asks me many hard questions which I have never talked about. About my mom, my family, my anxiety. I open up a bit, but I don't actually know how to verbalize much of what is going on in my mind and body.

The hospital doesn't allow access to the internet, and they restrict the television shows we watch. The type of shows are limited (no CSI or ER), and I have to go to bed at 10:00 p.m. I am only allowed to use the phone to call my father, which I do not do. Instead, I pace the halls.

One worker comes with a sheet for me to fill out. It is called "Create a list of ways you will remain safe upon being discharged from the hospital". As I am desperate to get out, I do what they ask and create a list of things they want to hear. The worker comes back and we talk about it.

"Now make a plan to talk to your dad about it."

Again, I do what they ask and say what they want to hear. I am desperate to get out and willing to do anything at this point.

At first, when I am admitted, they do not allow me to go to my room, yet they provide nothing to do otherwise. Later in the day, they finally allow me to go to my bedroom. I sit and look out at the parking lot from the windowsill.

There is nothing dangerous about me sitting there, as there is no way I could break through the window and jump from the building. It is more of a control thing. They want to tell me what I can and can't do. So, they tell me to get down from the window, again and again. Eventually they give up and I spend hours there, watching out of the window. I can tell when the shifts change. As I watch the workers leave and new workers arrive, the parking lot fills up and empties out.

My anxiety remains super high, and I constantly bounce my legs. They have taken away my journal, as it has a metal coil binding, instead they give me sheets of paper to write on. I see the psychiatrist a day after being admitted.

"I will not release you in this 'state'," he says.

"But I'm not going to take the pills!"

"No." he replies curtly, without any hint of compassion.

I know by 'state' he means mental state, but I take his words literally. I figure out how to suppress the anxiety and calm my body. My head is screaming, but my body is calm. For this reason, he cannot deny releasing me after a day, as I have no plans for suicide. They decide I will return to counselling with the local counsellor, and I am released into the care of my father. Before leaving, they permit me to shower in the shower room, which has a shower head about five feet off the ground, clearly designed for a child. I have to bend and lean over in order to wash my hair and body. It's just another sign that I don't belong here.

Immediately, when I get home from the hospital, I try to get out of the house. I pack for the weekend exercise with cadets. I do not dare tell anyone that I was in the hospital. I'm not sure why. Maybe I am embarrassed?

Feeling weak? I'm probably at least partially worried that my family will make fun of me. I can hear their voices in my head: "You loser." "No one cares if you live or die."

The weekend exercise is fun until one of my close friends, Sandy, hurts her back. The officers have not yet promoted Sandy. So, we leave her with the other cadets to iron and polish her uniform in order to increase her chances of promotion. A few of us are out on the back step, talking. We suddenly see an ambulance and fire truck pull up and we rush inside, wondering what the problem is. It turns out Sandy cannot move, and they have called an ambulance to take her to the hospital. We are all scared, and I feel particularly bad about leaving her to work on her uniform instead of socialising on the back step. Philipa, one of my other good friends, cries with worry. I wish I could cry too, but I am unable.

Philipa, is too upset to put more stress on her, thus I talk to my friend Kathy.

"I am trying to stop cutting," I share.

"I suspected you might cut," she responds.

Later that evening, we are relieved to find out that Sandy has sprained her back, but she has broken nothing. We are all relieved, but I feel guilty, wondering if I could have prevented this.

Journal Entry: Tuesday, September 27th, 2005

I am back at school but I don't care about class. I do not want to go back to the hospital. I'd rather die than go back. It screws up my life too much. I mean, look, I went the first time against my will and now I'm worse.

The idea of being back at school sucks. I'm all alone, and no one knows I was in the hospital. I can't rely on anyone else anyway, but I wish there was someone I could talk to… though I wouldn't talk to them, anyway. Going to the hospital was so traumatizing that I'll never do anything again that may make me go back. Going to the hospital just makes things worse.

Wednesday, September 28th, 2005

This morning, exactly two weeks after I am first admitted, I have a follow-up appointment with Evalyn.

"Tell me what went on while you were at the hospital?" Evalyn asks.

We talk about the hospital stay.

"I feel worse than I did before I went in there," I explained.

"How do you feel about the safety plan you made? Do you think you can commit to this safety plan?"

"Yes, I promise I won't hurt myself."

For some reason, no one thinks it is a good idea to take the pills from my locker at school. I am yet again incredibly depressed, and I've had enough. I don't want to do this anymore, and the world is better off without me. My family will be happier if I am gone. My useless self out of the way. The same day I make the promise to Evalyn, I sit out back behind the high school and take a bottle of Tylenol Extra Strength. I sit against the old brick wall. It is silent outside. No one is around. Three pills per sip is all I can swallow at once. I have several bottles of water, which allows me to take most of the bottle of Tylenol. As I wait for the pills to kill me, I am at peace. I assume I will slip into a coma and die like in the movies; however, I start to feel woozy and the lunch bell rings. I go to walk to my locker but feel dizzy, therefore I sit down on the cold hallway floor. My head pounds with the onslaught of students leaving classrooms, heading for lunch.

Then, I wait. I still assume I will pass out, slip into a coma, and die. But I do not. Instead, I now start to feel sick. Very sick. My stomach hurts and I panic.

"Ms. B" I look up with one hand on my stomach. The teacher stops. "I think I did something stupid," I say, starting to feel queasy.

"What's that?" she asks.

"I took a whole bottle of Tylenol."

"You need to go to the office. Can you make yourself throw up?" she asks, urgently.

"No."

She helps me up off the floor, takes my backpack and rushes me to the office, where they call an ambulance.

I am no longer really with this world. I seem to be in a distant, sort of out-of-body existence. The ambulance takes me back to the same hospital with the children's mental health unit.

"It's too late for charcoal," the ER doctor decides. "Let's give her some IV medications and let her throw up if she wants to."

I'm not aware of much during this time. They take me to the medical ward in a higher observation unit called Paediatric Intensive Care. I know they transfer me to the bed.

"Why would you do this to yourself?" a nurse says with compassion.

It takes twenty-four hours for my liver levels to come down.

"Okay, your liver levels are better now. I don't think you're going to have any permanent liver damage," the doctor explains to me while he stops in on his rounds.

My dad visits. He talks with the child psychiatrist just outside my door.

"Don't give her much attention or it will reward and reinforce her behaviour," the psychiatrist says to my father.

Because my levels improve, I am taken back to the children's mental health unit. They take away my clothes and replace them with hospital clothing. I must remove my shoes, and I am locked away again.

The staff on the children's mental health unit really push me to talk. I am resistant, but less so than last time. I break down a few times and finally have a call with my dad.

"Why won't you take me home?" I yell at him, "Why won't you just take me home with you? Instead of letting them lock me up in here!"

My dad comes to the hospital the next day during the day, and we have a long chat. He is not much better at communicating than I am, and it is awkward for both of us. One worker tries to help me relax so I can cry, which I do a bit. The unit social worker decides I should see one of their counsellors from the hospital. They arrange for my local counsellor to keep seeing me until I can start with the new counsellor at the hospital. The new counsellor is part of the Jones Clinic, which is a child and youth mental health program run by the hospital. It provides more intense counselling that the local youth centre counsellor can provide.

Chapter 3

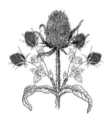

THE HOSPITAL DISCHARGES ME after one week, and as soon as I get home, I go to cadets. I do not want to be at home. Although it is Wednesday, I do not go in my uniform, as I am going to see my friends. No one called cadets last Wednesday when I took the pills, and one officer yells at me for not showing up without calling. It makes me feel terrible and lowers my mood more than it already is. I go out with Sandy, Philipa, and Kathy after cadets and we talk at a restaurant we frequently visit. I cry a bit (just a few tears down my cheek) and continue to cry when I get home until 3:00 a.m. On the one hand, I am upset that the officer's words affected me so much, but on the other hand, I am relieved to cry. It is one of the first times I have cried in years.

Previously, instead of crying, I would cut to avoid crying, but now I find myself wanting to cut so I cry.

I know I will get help from the new counsellor, but I am scared. I don't know if I'm supposed to be happy (at the prospect of help), sad (that I need help), or scared (with all the unknowns)? Maybe I can be all three at once. I am confused and frustrated. I was not happy to be going back to school in the first place, but now that I am back, I am feeling even worse.

I am not as far behind in English, but in Chemistry and Biology, I am too far behind to catch up. My teachers for those subjects allow me to skip the tests and assignments from unit one, but I still need to learn the material, as the later units build upon it. The work I need to catch up on is overwhelming. There is a lot of memory work and my memory is terrible. My brain doesn't want to work. I am sad and feel worthless. I hate feeling alone, yet I continue to isolate myself, as I feel there is no one there for me. I understand intellectually that there are people there for me, but emotionally I cannot reach out or connect.

Saturday, October 8th, 2005

I begin again with inner confusion. I am frustrated because I am confused and confused because I am frustrated. Everything sucks—school, home, family, friends, work, cadets, sports, and people in general. I don't really know when this all changed. I just know that today, right now, I enjoy nothing.

Journal Entry: October 8th, 2005

I am getting sick of people's fake offers for help. They say, "If you ever need it, I'm here for you," or "I'm always available if you need to talk". But they aren't, actually. They aren't

*available at 3:00 a.m. when I need to talk, or in the middle
of class. They aren't there when I am alone. They aren't there
when I have the urge to cut, but don't want to, so I feel like I
need/want to cry, but then I can't, which just makes me want
to cut even more. Or how I feel alone, even with my friends
or at school.*

I find some people will say they want to help. They
might even say they are available 'any time'. But the truth
is, although they mean well, they are not available when I
need them. And it doesn't matter anyway, as all too often
I feel alone, even when I am with people. It's a horrible
feeling when you are surrounded by a thousand other
students, yet feel utterly alone.

• • • ● • ● ● ● • •

Summer, 1995

As a child, I was pretty energetic. I had a good heart
and a nasty temper. My mom became a stay-at-home
mom who offered childcare, consequently, there were
always other children to play with. She was very
down-to-earth, encouraging us to be independent to
learn for ourselves. We had a lot of fun and did many
things that future generations would find shocking. We
all had bikes and would venture off for hours, to the
beaches, the conservation area, and to the river that sep-
arates Pickering from Toronto.

We had lots of adventures; we learned to play poker
with plastic chips, and we had a mock trial when my

brother's friend and I hung my mom's bra on the fence outside for all the parents to see when they picked up their children. My mom encouraged us to learn things for ourselves. One year, my mom and the kids tapped our two maple trees and boiled about 40 buckets of sap down to make a cup of maple syrup. Another time, we went out hunting on garbage day for things to take apart. We found a toaster oven and spent all day using my dad's tools to tear it apart and to learn how it works.

My mom's background was from India, my dad's family way back was British. My skin was a little darker than most of the kids in my dance class that I took when I was around eight years of age. I remember my mom raising hell about being told to buy a specific shade of nude tights for the dance recital that would look ridiculous on my darker skin. I can't remember what the outcome was.

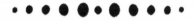

Journal Entry: Sunday, October 9th, 2005

I am understanding how much is wrong with me, both physically and mentally. I now can no longer keep up with others while they walk. My body moves too slowly. I stand up quickly and get dizzy or have a headache. I'm still 5'7 and 123 pounds and the nurses said that gaining weight will stop the dizziness. But I cannot eat, I don't have an appetite. I feel weak, both mentally and physically. Every time I try to socialize with my family, I get stressed. I am tired of feeling isolated, but feel unable to open up to even my closest friends. My dad seems to have forgotten all the communication stuff we talked about in the hospital. He agreed to ask me once in a while how I was feeling as I struggled to open up. But he doesn't ask, doesn't seem to care. I feel like things are back to the way they were and that we talk in code. I am now getting a bit optimistic about the therapy as I want to resolve these issues.

Despite the secret of my depression being out, I am not receiving help fast enough. My body and mind are moving slower and slower. I cannot walk as fast or think as clearly as the other students. It was bad before, but now it is worse. My father is not holding up his end of the bargain. The staff and I explained that I do not feel able to open up to him about how I am feeling without him asking. He agreed to ask me, but so far, he is not doing so. We talk in a kind of code, neither understanding exactly what the other is trying to get across. He appears unwilling, or perhaps incapable, of trying to meet my emotional needs.

"How are you?" He will occasionally ask half-heartedly.

"Fine," I reply, eyeing him carefully, trying to figure out if he really wants to know how I am doing.

"Good," he says

"Good," I respond back, and we go our separate ways.

Journal Entry: Wednesday, October 12th, 2005

*I don't understand my brain. I am frustrated with every-
thing yet I don't care all at the same time. It just makes little
sense. I cannot sleep at night. No matter what I do, I just can't
sleep. I'm tired during the day but can't sleep at night. I just
lay there awake, tossing and turning with my thoughts racing.
Therefore, I have to stay up doing something in order to not
go nuts. The thoughts are still there, but at least they're not as
bad when I'm occupied. To cope, I clean my room, over and
over.*

*I also want to care about school, but I don't. And that's
frustrating. I do things to try to make myself feel better, yet
when I do I feel worse after. This leads to me having to distract
myself from my thoughts or else I will start thinking about
dying again. So now I no longer want to get up to face the day.
Because, honestly, all I think about is death. So much that it
no longer scares me. And even when I think I find someone
who might understand and open up a little to them, I feel
worse after.*

I'm always cold, but in order to no longer feel cold, I
need to eat, which in turn makes me feel dizzy and sick.

I don't care about anything in life. I have this inner
sense of wanting to care, but I just can't make it happen. Part of that might be my logic telling me I'm not
worthless, but that's how I feel. I know I am a burden to
people I talk to. I take up their time, their thoughts, for
no reason. And because I am worthless, I am also alone;
everywhere, and especially at school.

My thoughts revolve around death, and I can think
of nothing else. I've tried distracting myself with music,
homework, cleaning, but nothing works. I'm scared that

I will cut again in order to get my mind off death. I don't want to do that, as I have not cut in two weeks and do not want to cut again. I want to bare my arms and join the swim team.

Thinking of all of this hurts my head. It makes me sad and I want to cry, but I can't. I'm unable to let myself cry even though I know I would feel better after. When I'm with other people, I can sometimes trick myself into thinking I feel better. I might smile or laugh a little, but the truth is I go home and feel worse. I wonder why I don't just stop going out. I can't rely on other people to make me smile, make me happy. I need to do it on my own.

I scared myself with what I did two weeks ago. What if I'd had more water? What if I'd had more pills? I'm torn. Part of me is thankful the water at school is not drinkable and therefore the number of water bottles I had limited how many pills I could take. But part of me also wishes I was dead. I don't know what part scares me more. Wanting to be dead or being confused.

I have screwed my life up so much. I'll never finish my English book by tomorrow, and I've screwed myself for the Biology Independent Study Unit. But then again, I don't care. I'm all alone at school, as I decided to do an extra year after all of my friends go on to post-secondary. I sit alone on the floor in a cold hall (which ironically is the warmest part of the entire school). It's only October, and I'm cold all the time. I'll never survive the winter. I'll have to wear long underwear under all of my clothes.

I'm worried that the cutting will come back, that I'm simply delaying the inevitable. I cut too deep before. My hand tingled, and it took an hour to stop the bleeding. What if one day I need stitches? Will they stick me back in the hospital? In the hospital they said cutting isn't a big deal (thank God), but what if a doctor overreacts? I can't spend more time there. I can't do that. It would destroy me. I really can't handle it. They need to help the people who can be helped. I'm hopeless. A lost cause. I can only feel okay for a short period, then I plummet. I don't know whether to expect a 'high' or a 'low'.

I've started thinking of a new way to kill myself. Maybe I could crash my car. Maybe take a bunch of aspirin to thin my blood, then slit my wrists. That way I would die and I wouldn't hurt anyone else like a car crash could. Gosh, I wish I was dead. I don't want to exist anymore.

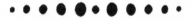

June, 1994

My mother was diagnosed with breast cancer. She was very young to have it, and it was not present in our family history, either. She previously had her spleen removed because of a platelet disorder called, (ITP) but they removed that long before she had children. When my mom got sick, I saw her as the person she was, not the illness. My aunt says I was the most empathetic of the kids. I guess that's why I eventually go into healthcare.

I remember very little of my mom being sick. I can recall visiting her in the hospital and eating her Jell-O. I remember watching TV on the little screen by her bed. I have very few other memories of her as a child, as I wasn't yet ten years of age when she died. The memories I hold are just short snapshots, such as playing with her wheelchair and running, pushing each other around the driveway in her wheelchair. It is a sweet memory, but not one that is directly about her.

I can remember being sick and being home from school. Our neighbour, Charlene, stopped by, and my mom made us each a cup of tea (mine was more milk and sugar than tea). I hid behind a book. I guess it embarrassed me to be home sick. I'm not sure.

Mom often had surprises for us if we had good behaviour. One day, I was called to finish the chocolate milk mixed with white milk. We used to call it 'marble milk' (although now that I'm older, I realize it was just a way to make the chocolate milk last longer).

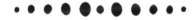

Thursday, October 13th, 2005

My father wants me to get a physical and books one with my doctor in a few weeks.

"I know you've never slept much, even when you were younger and you've always functioned. But now you're not sleeping much, and not functioning," as he explains his reasoning for the doctor's appointment.

It doesn't matter though; I don't care anymore. I hate everything and I want it all to end. Not so much die today, but end somehow. I hate feeling so worthless. Logic tells me I'm not, but I feel like it. It's a never-ending cycle. Feel like dying one day, feel not so bad the next day, feel like dying again the day after.

I miss the control that the cutting gave me. An ability to control the release of pain. Cut, bleed, pain relieved. All from blood, not tears.

Communication with my father is not going well. I feel like he is trying to order me around, forcing me to tell him how I feel (if he asks). All he has to do is ask nicely and genuinely. I would not say no. I would not lie to him. We planned how he could achieve this by going to Tim Hortons and talking with each other. But he doesn't want to do this. I have told him how to get me to talk with him, what words to use—he just shrugs it off. Instead, in the rare instances we do talk, he forces me to sit in the car outside Tim Hortons. I feel trapped there and although my muscles need to move, dizziness and headaches set in. I want to go home and never wake up again.

Journal Entry: Sunday, October 16th, 2005

I no longer enjoy work. I should. This is who I am, what I do. I love working with kids with special needs. But I don't enjoy anything anymore. I want to quit work but my dad does not approve. I honestly don't see the point of doing anything anymore. I don't see the point of being alive. I hate it. Why do anything? I want to quit work, quit everything, and die. I don't want to die by my own hand but it may end up being that way.

I'm going to stop letting my dad buy me dinner and stuff. It's too expensive. I'm not worth it. I can eat whatever there is at home if I decide to eat. Sometimes I just don't see the point. I bet this will be a bad week at school. This weekend was less-bad, therefore the week will be down.

I've come to realize there are doors in my head. It's a little hard to understand, but picture the movie Monsters Inc. *Remember all of the different doors leading to different bedrooms? Well it's the same idea. Logic behind one door, telling me one thing, like things are not my fault. Then there's the guilt door which opens and pours all over the logic door, making me feel that every bad thing that happens is my fault. I hate feeling like this all the time and I just want to die. I want to cry because I want to die so badly, but I can't. I can't cry anymore. I'm so confused. Some part of me remembers things I used to enjoy, then other parts of me just don't care and can't enjoy, so it doesn't matter.*

Journal Entry: Tuesday, October 18th, 2005

I don't want to do anything today. I want everything to end. I'd rather be dead. I want to take some aspirin and slit my wrists. Or maybe take some sleeping pills and drown in the bathtub. I don't care anymore. I just want to be at home in bed. I just want everything to end. Why won't it end? I want to kill myself but I said that I wouldn't. So now I'm just waiting to be in that car crash, to be hit by that lightning bolt. I just want to be dead. Maybe I should piss off some gangsters so that they'll come shoot me. I just want it all to end. Please. Someone. Make it end.

I might call my dad after this class and ask him to sign me out for the rest of the day. I just want to go home. At least there I can sleep and hope that I will never wake up. It would be so nice for everything to just end. Dead. Gone. No more. Just take a blade and slit the wrists. Or take a gun and shoot myself in the head. Something. Anything. I just want to be dead. How nice would it be to no longer feel? It would be amazing. Well it would be nothing, because I wouldn't be able to feel amazing. I wish for nothingness. I wish I was dead.

My guidance counsellor suggests maybe I should focus on getting my English credit with 2 easier credits so that I can graduate and get out of high school. Then I can go to college. She also thinks I should talk to the board psychologist to help with the motivation. I don't think she realizes <u>why</u> I'm not motivated. Why care about schoolwork if I no longer care about living? I just want to be dead, so what is the point of getting credits? I don't want to be here. I don't want to exist.

I can't see how I can possibly get better. The only way I can see it getting better is to have everything end. To Die. Be gone. No more. Nothingness. I hate being here. The idea of a college diploma, then university when I am ready, makes sense in some ways, for someone who cares. But I just want to be dead. I wish I hadn't told Evalyn last time when I took the pills. Then I would be dead and not going through this. I can't wait until the day comes that I finally die. I just can't wait. I really hope that therapy will help, but I'm not really expecting it to. I'm too low, too down. There's only one option left - Death. But I said that I wouldn't do it myself. I'll just have to wait until death comes to me.

Later in October, I have a doctor's appointment and in November my new therapy starts at the hospital. I wonder if it's worth it to stick around just to fail again. I don't want to fail again. Maybe I should just slit my wrists.

I know which course I would drop if I could: Biology. I'm just too screwed for it. I understand it, but I can't memorize it like this. Memory is just another thing for me to fail at. I suck so badly. Oh well. Once death comes, it won't matter anymore. People say to take life as a challenge. What if you don't want to be alive? You don't want to take that challenge? I am sick of the big, bad, ugly, dark low that controls my life.

• • • ● • ● ● • • •

Wednesday, October 19th, 2005

My appointment with my family doctor is this morning. He says he will give me a prescription for Ativan for sleep at the end of the appointment. He asks about how I am feeling, how long I was in the hospital, then gives me the prescription and mentions about getting me something for my mood.

Next, I go to my appointment with Evalyn, then to the blood lab. My dad takes me to Denny's, where I try to eat some breakfast food. We go to my school to drop off the psychologist's form and my dad signs me out for the rest of the day. At home, I prepare my uniform for cadets but in the end decide not to go, as I can't handle the stress.

Journal Entry: Wednesday October 19th, 2005

The first time I tried the Ativan, I realized it is a crazy medication. The first 20 minutes I feel nothing, then after 20-40 minutes I start to feel something, then sensory stuff happens. First mild stuff, then at about 1hr 20mins I notice that if I shake my head the music and lights pulse. At the close to 2 hour mark, it finally starts to calm me down. I am still easily distracted, but I am more relaxed.

Journal Entry: Monday, October 24th, 2005

This is just so confusing. There are some days when I care, and some days when I just don't care, and some days when I just don't know. There are so many things going on in my head, twisting and turning my thoughts until I no longer recognize them.

I try to talk to my dad but he doesn't understand that I'm tired of fighting. These meds are my last resort and if they don't work or get delayed again, I will kill myself. I'm on my last straw here. And I don't know who I can talk to about it. I don't have an appointment with Evalyn, plus I worry that she'd have to put me in the hospital again. Teachers are teachers, they don't know how to handle this kind of stuff. And it's not their responsibility. I just want to go somewhere and cry, but our school sucks and there's nowhere to go.

I would love to have a list that says who I can talk to and what about. I don't know how to talk to people. Have I scared away the ones I have spoken small bits to? I just don't know. I hate all this. I'm ready to give up. No more of this challenge crap. I'm done. Spent. I want to say goodbye to the world. I'm fed up and want it all to end.

What's right? What's wrong? What's normal? I have no sense to differentiate. I've always assumed these voices in my head were normal. What if they aren't? What if I tell someone and they make them go away? I would be even more alone. What about the cutting? Is it killing me or keeping me alive? Everything is so twisted in my mind.

• • • ● • ● ● • • •

Wednesday, October 26th, 2005

Today I see my family doctor again. He gives me a prescription for a drug called Clonazepam to help me sleep and a sample for a drug called Effexor XR to start tomorrow. It is a starter sample kit. I wonder if he is giving it to me because he thinks it is the best medication for me or because he has the samples in his office, but I don't care enough to question it.

When I get back to school later in the morning, I meet with the board psychologist before going to English for part of the class before going to my appointment with Evalyn.

"I have my first appointment with Amelia, my new therapist at The Jones Clinic, tomorrow and I'm really worried," I say to Evalyn.

"Try to not worry, breathe, and TALK. Say everything that comes to your mind and don't make it hard on her," Evalyn encourages me.

I also quit my job today and my dad is okay with it. My boss is pretty good about it too.

My dad still does not stick to the talk schedule we established in the hospital where he is supposed to ask me, at least on Tuesdays, Thursdays, Saturdays, and Sundays. But those four days he must ask. In the hospital we had talked about me being unable to take up his time and that he needs to ask me how I am feeling. How my day went. I need him to engage and follow the schedule. I'm talking to him a bit more freely, but I still need those four sit-down talks. He says it's always a good time to talk, but it's not.

Summer, 1995

My mom and her sister Tina were very close. One time, my aunt came to visit and told me she had a present for me.

"Is it underwear?" (I'm not sure why I guessed that.)

"No," she said.

A few hours later, my aunt gave me a pack of underwear, and I lost it. Total meltdown. My mom was so mad at me. I don't think I was upset that I got underwear, but that they had assured me it was not. My mom forgave me, though, and a few days later she gave me a Tamagotchi toy.

"Here you go Liz. I had already purchased this for you the other day, but I didn't give it to you because of your behaviour," my mom said as he handed the toy to me.

She was very fair like that. There was always a reason for her treatment with us, and she would always forgive.

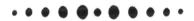

Summer, 1999

I had other meltdowns throughout the years. At one point, I locked my siblings in the pool yard. I don't know why; I must have been mad at someone about something. Our parents weren't home and my older sister was watching us. My brother had to hop the pool fence to get the key from inside the house. Another time, I put the leg of a stool through my bedroom door (then, realizing my mistake, I tried to hide it with duct tape).

Thursday, October 27th, 2005

I'm getting nervous and especially worried about my first impression with Amelia. Today is a better day, partially because I dropped Chemistry and Biology. Now I will do a co-op at a local elementary school in their kindergarten class. This means I help out the teacher and learn how to work with kids. I prefer this idea to the science courses, but it's a lot of responsibility that I'm not sure I'm ready to take on.

Amelia seems to be nice and understanding when I meet her. I think I can work with her, which is a bit of a relief. I want things to work out because I really believe this is my last chance. Having to try again is too much for me.

Chapter 4

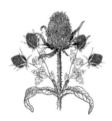

TUESDAY, NOVEMBER 1ST, 2005

Today I see the hospital social worker for our first true session (not the meet & greet). I have just started the Effexor. We talk a bit about my mom and how I feel, my grief and where it hurts.

"Where do you hurt?" Amelia asks. "Where in your body do you hurt? Can you draw me a picture of where you hurt?"

I colour a picture that shows the area of hurt in the centre of my chest.

"So, how are you feeling now?" she asks, at the end of the session

"I feel I need to cut," I tell her, trying to be honest.

"Let's bring your father in here, okay?" she tells me, making it sound like I have a choice in the matter.

"Hi Mr. Grace. Liz has shared with me that she feels a need to cut," she explains to my father as he sits next to me in the small office. "I need you to take away her razors and watch over her."

"Okay." He says. He never says much.

I am present for their conversation, I am concerned. I know, without my blades, I can't survive. They can't keep taking them from me. I was only going to cut my arm, not my wrist. The feeling of relief is what I need. I need my blades to survive. I cut to survive. If I can't have them, I won't survive. I am tired of voices yelling things. I am tired of doors. I'm tired of everything.

I go home and go to my room, but my father doesn't come to take the blades. I'm not sure how long I am there before I take a razor to my arm. I feel the water calling and I am scared but not sure of what. The calling is like a sweeping, unearthly feeling that runs through my body and mind. It is telling me I need to go to the lake, which is less than one kilometre away. This time when I cut, I hit the brachial artery in my left elbow, and suddenly the blood is shooting across the room. I am scared and don't know what to do, as the bleeding is not stopping.

"Dad!"

When he comes in, I say, "I think I cut too deep."

"Brian!" my dad calls out to my brother.

I'm not aware of much. My brother is a paramedic student; therefore, he knows to keep pressure on the wound while my dad drives me back to the hospital.

At the hospital, they put me in a quiet room. I cannot talk, and while the doctor stitches my wounds, I'm looking at dragons on the wall and ceiling. A red one and a blue one. Just like Mushu, the dragon in the animated film *Mulan*. Of course, I cannot tell anyone I see them, as I cannot talk from the shock and dissociation of the whole incident.

As I cannot talk, they decide I am not enough of a risk to need to be hospitalized, and they send me home. I spent the next two days in bed, not talking and not eating. I must get up to go to the bathroom, but I'm not very aware. The lake begins to call me again. It is calling me with its essence. It feels like it's pulling my soul.

My father no longer knows what to do with me. Thursday morning, he forces me to drink an Instant Breakfast and calls the social worker at the hospital. They decide it is time to put me back in the hospital. I'm not sure how I get there. I assume my dad drives me. We wait for hours in the ER. There are no beds in the children's ward, consequently I am placed on the adult ward with extra supervision at first. They try to get me to eat a cold pizza, but I'm too spaced out. My mind isn't focusing on the here and now. I'm thinking about the lake and monsters and focusing on the unworldly sensations going through my body. They sit me outside the nurses' station and a nurse tries to talk to me.

"I have a friend who has a daughter... My friend's daughter is ten years old and her mom is dying of cancer. Do you have any advice on how I can help the little girl?" the nurse asks.

But I am afraid that there is a monster hunting me down, sent by the lake. I do not want to talk, as talking will alert it to my location. I try to write in my journal (which I am allowed to have on the adult ward) but she refuses to let me write to her.

"No. don't write it down, tell me, aloud, how I can help her. Use your voice."

I try, but I get so worked up. I begin to hyperventilate, wring my hands and hit myself. The nurse brings me to bed, where I lay for a while, before I get up and bang the back of my head on a pillar. I realize that the nurse was trying to trick me into talking, therefore revealing my location to the monster. If she really cares about what I have to say, she will let me write. This stresses me out because she made me talk. I get up, go into the hall, and see the monster. I shove it away, only to realize that it was actually another patient. When I realize she is not the monster, my anxiety increases. Now all I can do is bang my head on the corner of a pillar in the corner of my room to get the lake to stop calling me.

The nurses stop me from banging my head and I am put back to bed. But later that night, the water calls again. I feel the chill of the lake calling me, and I am convinced it is nearby, so I get up out of bed. I must get out of here. I have to get to the water. It is calling me, or else the monster will come get me.

My fear of the monster is reaching a new high. It is early in the morning, but I must silence anything that may call him. There is a man next door, and I can hear him snoring.

"Shut up! Shut up! Shut up!" I shout at him. He needs to be quiet, as he is calling the monster. By now, it doesn't matter if my yelling will call the monster. That snoring already did.

Before the monster arrives, I know I must escape. I try to kick down the (locked) emergency doors and sneak onto the elevator. I am pacing around the unit, trying to figure out how to get out.

"Come with me. Sit. Sit in this chair," a nurse says sternly as she puts me in a kind of chair with a tray to keep me away from the doors, but being a nimble seventeen-year-old, I can hop out of it easily.

I am not staying in this hospital. I need to get out before I am taken by the monster.

The staff decide to put me in the isolation room, which is in the children's unit. That, however, just escalates my distress, as now I am locked in a room within a unit.

"Hey! Let me out! Let me out of here!" I yell, I scream. "Please, please let me out of here. Please, let me out. Please!" I bang on the windows, hoping to break them down. "You don't understand. He's coming. I have to get out of here!"

The staff does nothing, just leaves me there, hoping I will calm down. They don't see how they are making the situation worse, escalating my anxiety and flight response. Eventually, they realize I'm not calming down in the room, and that my yelling is waking up the children in the unit.

Someone unlocks and opens the door. There are several security guards and they are grabbing me. I am forced out of the room, back into the adult ward, and into my room. They must have moved the lady next to me, as she does not appear to be in the room. Someone has attached the baby blue restraints to my bed and the staff give one last attempt to calm me down, which does not work, as the security guards are holding me forcefully. Again, I am still fearful of the monster. I try to escape, at which point the security guards and nurses decide they need to forcefully restrain me.

I am literally fighting for my life. They are not only physically assaulting me with their strength, but they are tying me up, restricting my freedom, and making me easy prey for the monster.

Author's note:
Let me pause here and explain being restrained. It's not like the movies, where they wrap you in a straitjacket and put you in a white padded room. No, first security guards and sometimes nurses tackle you. They hold you down on a bed while you are distressed, and lock you into four-point restraints (wrists and ankles). If you don't calm down at this point, they take a shockingly large needle, pull down your pants (possibly in front of other staff and patients), stab it in your butt cheek, and chemically restrain you until you don't know up from down. Meanwhile, while all this is happening, **they tell you it's for your own good.**

When you wake up, you are calm, yet still restrained. They have an arbitrary amount of time that you are supposed to be calm in the restraints before they let you out. I don't know whose guideline this is, but they've obviously never been tackled, strapped to a bed, medicated, and then told they have to continue to stay calm before they are released. Who can stay calm for that? It's barbaric. I can't think of any situation where it is acceptable for a person to be held down and have things done to them against their will. It should be banned. Even a prisoner would have access to human rights advocates and a lawyer.

I am not sure what happens next, and I assume they have given me a drug. When I wake up, there are several nurses in my room. I lock eyes with one and can't let go. A wave of distress washes over me every time she looks away. I feel she is my only hope. If I can just get her to save me, I will be okay.

I am not sure how long all of this goes on. It feels like hours to me. All this stress and commotion upsets my bowels, which have been backed up for days due to not eating and drinking.

"Can you let me up? I need to go to the bathroom. I need to go. I need you to let me up, so I can go into the bathroom! Please?"

After asking several times to go to the bathroom and realizing I need to force myself to calm down if I'm going to be released and not crap the bed, I force myself to shut down. I give in and accept that the monster is going to get me, take me to the lake, and torture me forever.

"Please, I need to go to the bathroom." I ask urgently. They release me and I barely make it to the toilet before my bowels let loose.

The ward psychiatrist must have heard about the incident, as he visits me.

"I'm going to take you off of this antidepressant," he says with my chart in his hands.

"Please, put me back on it. I cannot go any longer without an antidepressant. I am too ready to die," I request. He listens and puts me back on it.

There is a lady on the adult ward who screams and screams. I am worried that she is calling the monster and I scream back at her. This results in me being restrained again, although this time I do not remember as much.

Shortly after that, I am transferred to the children's ward, where I continue to be drawn to the water. I pace the unit, taking every opportunity to escape. Several more times, I am restrained. The pacing is because the monster is coming and the lake is calling.

"Stop pacing," a staff member snaps at me.

I turn around, grab their wrists, and pin them to the wall. I'm not entirely aware I am doing it and certainly not realizing I am doing it to them. But yet again, there I am, getting tackled by security guards, strapped to a bed. I am told to stay calm before they will let me out.

Over the six weeks I am in the hospital, I am restrained thirteen times, and it feels like I am getting punished for being afraid. My spirit is broken. There is no attempt by the staff to de-escalate. They immediately call security, wrestle me to my room, and tie me down any time I start to escalate. I try everything I can to get out. My hands and wrists are so small that I can slip my hands out of the restraints. But they lock the restraints magnetically, hence I cannot remove the ankle ones. They think it is a game to me, that I enjoy being strapped down. Rest assured; it is not. Most people would re-evaluate their hypothesis after the first three times, but the staff continue with their belief that I am acting out so they can restrain me for attention. However, in reality, I am fighting for my life. And doing that includes doing whatever I have to do to get out. Sometimes there are other pieces to the puzzle, like when I am in restraints and see my room on fire.

"There's fire! Fire in my room," I shout. "Please let me out. I'm going to die in here!"

They ignore me.

Only to say, "You're fine! Stop yelling!"

They don't understand that I am literally facing my death from more than one threat. It's kind of ironic that I am fighting for my life, given I also want to die. Perhaps I do not want to be forced to live a life I do not want to live while being strapped to a bed.

When all of this starts, I am started on an antipsychotic called Zyprexa Zydis. I think it is the trendy medication at the time, as every patient on the children's ward seems to be on it. The medication is a yellow disc that dissolves in my mouth. It tastes funny, and if eaten within a few minutes of certain foods, I get a disgusting taste in my mouth and want to vomit. It also makes me hungry, like *starving*. In the six weeks I am in hospital, I gain a ton of weight. I go from 123 pounds to probably 135 pounds (a nine percent increase in just six weeks). For a teenager, this is a huge amount of weight to gain, and I am distressed by the changes to my body. None of my clothes fit when I am eventually discharged to go home.

During this hospital stay, someone, somewhere, decides that I'm not actually sick.

"She just wants attention."

So, all the staff start telling me this.

"You aren't sick."

"You're making this up."

"You just want attention."

"You can control this yourself."

I am told these things, over and over and over. No one cares that the water is calling me or that nobody in their right mind would put themselves in a situation where they are going to be restrained, yet there I am. To them, it is just a matter of me stopping the behaviour that I am choosing to exhibit.

They permit me to bring some things from home (like socks and underwear) when I have a pass home. I secretly hide a shaving razor in my bag in my locker, just in case I need to cut. They do not find it when I come back from a pass. I am not bringing the razor to be bad or break the rules. Cutting saves me. I still do not have coping strategies to deal with the pain inside of me, and cutting is the only way I know how. I feel safer knowing I have a razor in my bag, even if they lock it up in a locker.

Sometimes I can feel the monster and try to distract myself with writing. I can see him lurking in the shadows, but I know the staff will tell me he isn't real and to stop vying for attention. Often now, I wake up in the middle of the night fearful and trying to escape. I sleepwalk and try to steal the staff ID badges and get out the doors, which results in me being restrained often at night. There are voices constantly telling me to run from the monster. I keep this to myself.

I want to avoid being told, "You're just making it up to get attention," by the staff again.

The staff are so convinced of this idea that it is a behaviour for attention that I begin to believe it myself. I'm not really sick. I'm not really having these visions or experiences. The voices are my own. I'm just wanting attention from my dad. We come up with the idea to make a list of things I can do when I feel these things.

"You are in control and you can stop this behaviour," some staff member tells me. I tell myself I can do this by doing things like doing a puzzle, listening to music, or colouring.

I have so many things going on in my head, one of which is this concept of doors—every door in my mind holding a distinct feeling or experience or even a command (like 'grab the keys') that I have to do. Staff won't understand if I tell them I go for the unit door because the lady behind the door in my mind tells me I have to.

I try to do what they ask to make myself better. I tell myself to 'act normal', and I am trying to follow their rules to behave, and I decide to let the staff know that I have the razor so they can take it away. While I am not put in restraints for this, they revoke my visitor privileges and I am not permitted visitors at night. I am so confused. I do what they ask, yet I get punished. It confuses my sense of reality and I stop understanding what I am and am not supposed to do.

The medications must be working in some respect, as I am no longer overly suicidal. I do, however, continue to worry about the monster and water calling me. I'm sure the doctor at this point doesn't know what to do with me. My emotions are on a roller coaster. They were before this hospitalisation, but they are now worse, as I want to be dead. I fear that I'm going to be kidnapped and tortured. I am also being tackled and assaulted several times a week by staff and security. Throughout all this, I am told this is all a behaviour that is 100% in my control.

Finally, the doctor sets up a phone call between myself and a program in a nearby town. The program deals with people with emotional problems. It is a residential program in a big house with twelve patients, all with emotional problems. Patients reside there Monday to Friday. It is in the community and not a hospital. I will be eighteen soon and therefore qualify to go. The intake worker talks to me over the phone, and it becomes clear that I just have to tell them what they want to hear to get myself out of the hospital. I don't want to lie, but my hands are tied.

"I am just doing all of this for attention," I tell the doctor. "And I would like to attend the residential program."

To do that, they must take me off all of my medications before I can start in January. The last piece is that I must

tell my dad that my behaviour was all for attention. I do
not want to do this. I do not want to lie, and I know
it will probably hurt him. But I am left with no choice.
My father's wedding to Janet is tomorrow, and if I am
not there, the family will move on without me.

"Dad," we sat down at a table. "I think, I've realized,
all this… it's just to get your attention" I speak this lie.
One I so desperately do not want to tell. Given the
circumstances, I have no choice. And he believes me.

Chapter 5

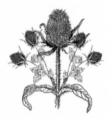

T HE NEXT DAY, finally home, I go to Sears to find
something suitable for the wedding. Nothing fits
me in my closet because I have put on so much weight.
I only have a bit of money in my bank account to buy
something to wear. I settle on a nice-looking red sweater
with black dress pants.

They hold the wedding on a winter evening, and I
pretend to be happy for my dad and Janet. In some ways
I am; I want my father to be happy and have someone
in his life. But I can't help feeling like an afterthought.
They were going to go ahead with the wedding, with
or without me. My sister, at the University in Sudbury,
had to take a bus down this morning and a midnight bus
back tonight because she has an exam tomorrow. They
had changed the wedding date once already because
it was more favourable for one of her daughters, but

apparently my mental health or my sister's exam are not important enough reasons.

Things do not start off well at home. First thing, before the wedding, Janet asks us if we can put clean sheets on my father's bed before they come home from the wedding. Janet has been to our home many times by now and should know my father has not gotten rid of a single item which belonged to my mother. She should know that the closet is still full of my mother's things and her side of the bed still has my mom's stuff on it. Thankfully, they decide to stay in a hotel for the first night.

Once my father and Janet are married, Janet immediately moves into our house with her son. They give my room, my sanctuary, to her son, and I am forced back into sharing a room with my thirteen-year-old sister. My mental health worsens from this, and Janet ends up being the one (through no fault of her own) to go through my mother's belongings because my father does not do it himself. He puts her in a bad situation. It is not her responsibility nor place to make room for herself by removing my deceased mother's belongings.

At home, I am so out of sorts and lost. I no longer have a room, which means I no longer have a place of my own to relax and calm down. I am now always on edge and cannot relax in my sister's messy room. As I have gained twelve pounds while in the hospital, none of my clothes fit, so I have very little to wear. I decide I need to lose weight and will start with a two-day water cleanse, then switch to low-cal foods. I don't want to be fat anymore, and I'm disgusted with myself when I have to buy size large pants. When I break my diet and eat and eat, I feel like I lose control. I want to throw up but don't/can't. I am bad and I'll eat nothing tomorrow.

For New Year's Eve, my boyfriend's family throws a party. I feel distanced from everyone. I don't know how I will handle the changes and being distant from my friends when I go to Beacon House. I want to kill myself again, but I won't. I wish I could, it would be so relieving.

My dad is building me a room in the basement, but it is slow, and I will share a bedroom with my sister for a long time. I cry myself to sleep often. Sometimes because I need my space, sometimes because I am worried about the Beacon House program—the residential program a few towns over for adults with emotional disturbances—and sometimes because I feel worried about being away from my friends. My life is falling apart. I am just a sick little girl, and I'm not even that anymore. I'm fat and I need to lose weight.

Sometimes I wonder if maybe I'd rather be back in the hospital and just let the voices take over. It takes everything I have to not act on what they say (like to go to the lake). I think about how any actions that my mind wants to take will hurt my dad or my family, and so I take the punishment my mind gives me for not acting. I refuse to hurt anyone anymore.

I feel little of anything anymore now that they have stopped the medications in order for me to attend the Beacon House program. I still feel like cutting. Sometimes I feel like I should cut to take away the anxiety and other times I feel like I should cut to purposely feel the anxiety. It makes no sense, which is evidence of my twisted brain.

My last night before Beacon House, I feel nothing. Not excited, not sad. I know I should feel anxious, but I don't even feel that. When they took me off the medication, I completely lost interest in school. I feel like a blank canvas, ready to be painted. I never have been anything, and I never will be anything again. It's just the way it is. I wish I could feel something. Even pain would be better than nothing at all.

In order to attend this residential program for people with emotional disturbances on January 3rd, 2006, I have to taper off all my medications. Absolutely everything psychiatric. I may not be on an antidepressant, anything for anxiety or sleep, and no antipsychotics. Patients may have physical medicines for blood pressure etc., but nothing psychiatric.

I will sleep there during the week, then go home on the weekend. I meet privately with the staff (who I don't think are actual therapists), and they want me to talk about my feelings. In group they also want us to open up, but we may not comfort each other, ever. I try to pass a box of Kleenex to another patient when she cries, and I am immediately told to stop. If she wants a Kleenex, she has to get it herself, because if I hand it to her, she is getting attention. I don't see this as attention-seeking; I see this as a chance for compassion, and I don't understand what kind of program promotes the removal of compassion. It blows my mind and I feel even more alone, hopeless, and it deepens my desire to die.

I find it hard to relate to the other patients. They are all older, mostly women. They talk about moms in groups, but not remembering much of my mother, I have nothing to contribute. I worry about sharing a room at night with a stranger. At home, I'm in my sister's room. It's her room, not mine. But here I am to share a room with another lady. Since I am also not permitted any sleeping medications, I worry about sleep walking that led to being restrained in the hospital. Will it happen again?

I am a picky eater and find myself unable to eat many of the meals provided, cooked in turns by the patients in the program. Since I am no longer at home or at school for twelve weeks, I have had to give up cadets, school, and dragon boat racing. These are the things that make me 'me', and I am even more lost and unsure of myself. I try to run daily to keep up my fitness and lose weight from the Zyprexa. My body is in pain, but I push through. So few of my clothes fit and I want to get back in shape before I have to return to school. I run down to the water a few kilometres away. It is winter, cold, and the water is choppy. It matches my internal feelings.

The psychiatrist of the program assesses me and determines that I do not have Borderline Personality Disorder (the prevailing diagnosis of the others in the program).

After a week, I am ready to give up. What kind of life is worth living if we withhold compassion? A life where I am constantly told that I am the problem, not the environment of my home life? At home I did not learn how to handle my emotions, did not learn how to grieve, and my father did not show me enough respect to tell me things instead of assuming I can mind read. My home environment after my mom's death did not include siblings caring about each other and did not include discipline or routine. Did not include learning life skills like how to maintain a clean house, maintain the outside of the house, or how to cook. Why would I want to work for the rest of my life to suppress my emotions while pretending to open up? The water calls, and I think, *what is the point?*

I feel like crying and miss my family.

"Go be with the other patients," my dad tells me, when I speak to him on the phone.

Now I am even more alone. I try to do what they ask, which is to talk to them when feeling poorly. I tell the staff what I have now learned to believe to be true of myself.

"I don't really want to get better and I just want the attention." I tell her, "I think I isolate myself for attention."

They have drilled this into my head as the reason for my episodes, and my mind is accepting it as the truth. I talk with some of the other patients, and I talk about how I plan everything and keep my control by planning. My routines, my conversations, they run through in my head a million times before it happens for real.

The therapist I work with talks to me about the cutting.

"Show me where you have cut yourself," she demands. She wants to see my scars. "You need to be honest."

I am confused—I thought I was being honest, but now I am second guessing myself. Can I be honest? I am so conflicted by what's going on in my head that I don't even know what being honest means.

"Liz, do you want to be here? Liz, do you want to get better?"

Part of me doesn't want to, as part of me wants to be dead. Will all of me want to get better by the end of this program?

"Are you going to be stuck back in the hospital?"

As we sit in silence, I begin to think that it will probably be true. I will probably end up in the hospital again.

"When you get better, you will want to go back to school and want to do stuff again."

I think she might be trying to be encouraging. I get confused in my own thoughts; do I want to get better?

During some puzzle time, one participant gives me some wise words "You can always go back to being sick but you should take this chance to get better," she puts a couple of interlocking pieces together.

So, I stick with that idea and say it to myself over and over.

My worker insists I have a personality disorder, that I am irresponsible, have bad coping skills, poor relationships, and difficulty expressing emotions and resolving conflict. This is strange for me to hear, as I have always been the responsible person, not the irresponsible one. I have always been the mediator. However, I accept her opinion as fact, as surely, she knows what she is talking about. I'm not sure how she makes this judgement after knowing me less than a week.

The first time I meet with the 'therapist', we talk about how I will introduce myself to the group. How will I talk about my mom, my dad remarrying, my cutting, my poor coping, my controlling, wanting to be sick, doing poorly in school even though I'm very smart? I am supposed to tell the group that I don't know what to say, but I welcome questions. It doesn't matter if I do or not.

In the program, there are various groups, one of which is Addictive Behaviours. They tell me cutting, hitting, even avoiding making decisions are all addictive behaviours, and these are all my problems to fix. I tend to teeter on the fence and let decisions be made for me. Even coming here, I didn't make that decision. My dad did.

I witness these 'behaviours' from the Addictive Behaviours group in other patients in the program. Most are ladies in late middle-age, probably around fifty, and a few men, but no one is young like me. There is one lady with the attitude that everyone is out to get her and no matter how much we reassure her, she won't believe it. I learn that if I don't start putting myself first, I will get nowhere.

The voices are still there, but I have been telling myself they are just in my head. When the staff announces they are considering allowing in patients who are on medications, I am torn. On one hand, how can they allow some people to have meds when it was a requirement for the rest of us to be off? My meds helped me a lot, but now that I am off them, I see maybe I can live without them.

The group gets to me again. I look at the other patients and foresee a terrible life for myself. I think of that Kleenex box, where I even may not give or receive that tiny bit of compassion lest I be seeking attention. I try to talk to the staff, but unfortunately, I am brushed off, told I am being dramatic, and left with my hopelessness. Life isn't worth living if it is like this, and I take an overdose of aspirin.

I am sitting on the floor swallowing pills when someone walks into the room.

"You are seeking attention," I am told and again taken to the hospital.

This time they give me charcoal, then admit me to the psych floor. The charcoal is a black, chalky liquid that I am forced to drink but quickly throw up. In the psychiatric ward, I share a room with a woman who believes Jesus is talking to the world through her. I have never been a religious person, but I see how much it comforts her to believe this.

I regret taking the pills and I wish I could have held it together for twelve weeks. Maybe it would have changed my life. Janet makes an effort to visit me, and we talk.

"We suspected something might have been going on, but we had expected he would tell us if he was dating someone seriously."

After she leaves, I write on my hands the words "Normal", "Get Well", "Be Good", "WWDWYTD" (What Would Dad Want You to Do?). A constant reminder to be good, that it is all behaviour, and it is my decision to control it.

Being good becomes the focus of my life. I force myself to be the good child they want and not allow myself to be bad and out of control. I reflect on my crash out of the program and feel as though I really don't know what caused it. The psychiatrist is the same doctor from the other hospital and the hospital therapy centre. He offers to refill the Effexor, but I do not feel that it helps. He puts me back on the Zyprexa, and I will try an alternative antidepressant in the hopes that I will get back my motivation for school. I don't want to be a dropout.

I am ready to leave the hospital, and the psychiatrist discharges me, but my father will not take me home. I am sure that I know when I am safe and when I am not. My father does not believe me. He wants me to get therapy in the hospital, but such a thing does not exist. He does not understand what it is like to be in the hospital, how it makes me worse. Staying in the hospital would make me lose my life, my friends, my family. He doesn't tell me why he won't take me home, but I assume he is as tired of the mental illness as I am. I expect Janet has also played a role in this decision, as she has never liked me, and I can do nothing right in her eyes. I worry I will end up on the street.

I am discharged from the hospital, and with nowhere to go, I end up in a crisis bed/shelter in a mental health group home, technically homeless. Beacon House will not take me back, saying I am too impulsive for the program. Essentially, I am too sick; my behaviour is too extreme for them, the program for people with extreme behaviour problems. I'm not sure where they expect me to find help.

I worry about the instability of a shelter and how that will impact my ability to be good. I am offered up to three nights in the shelter, then I am on my own. That first night in the crisis bed/shelter in the group home, I pray to Jesus. I have nothing to lose, so I try it.

I find no comfort in it. I tell myself I am calmer and that it is nice to know that God is always with me and I am never alone. I try with all my heart to believe it, but in the back of my mind, I do not.

I worry about what will happen if my dad and Janet don't take me home. I won't be able to afford food, shelter, and trips to see Amelia. I wonder what I'm going to have to give up and what kind of hellhole I will end up living in. Regardless of their decision, I am determined to survive. I will show them I am good; show them I am capable. In the morning, after not sleeping well, my jaw is so sore. I must be clenching it, but that is the least of my worries at present.

I make a list to show I am good and in control. I write my signs of distress (not eating, not sleeping, isolating myself, jumbled thoughts, feeling very sad/depressed, doors and voices in my head, feeling of the water calling) and things to tell myself (don't hurt Dad, be strong) and I keep trying the "God is with you" mantra. When I need help, I will call the crisis line and see Amelia regularly. I also write a list of things to do when feeling 'bad' (read a book, watch a movie, listen to music, dance, volunteer at the school, and write in my journal).

After a few days, my dad and Janet say they want me to go into a group home. We talk to the Canadian Mental Health Association about supportive housing, but there is a wait list until mid-summer at least. There are no openings anywhere, for which I am thankful. The group home I am at has all double rooms, with no privacy for any residents. It would be a terrible place to live; however, it means I am yet again without a roof over my head when my three days are up. Dad and Janet reassure me I won't end up in a shelter, but I don't believe them, as I'm already here in one. If they don't take me home, where will I go? They don't understand what it's like and how horrible it would be to live among people, but still be alone.

I make another plan. I focus on how I will be an average teen with an average lifestyle. I will go back to school, go back to cadets, get a job, see my friends, get back into sports, and do fun things with the family. For school, I am going to stay motivated, finish my courses, and make new friends. I will get to bed earlier so I can get up earlier and pack and prepare a lunch daily. My obstacles to this plan include my emotions, for which I will go to counselling and focus on coping by being a regular teen with regular reactions to the regular world.

The next day, my dad and Janet take me to Tim Hortons to talk. They say they will always be there for me and agree to take me home.

Chapter 6

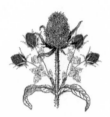

M ID-JANUARY 2006

Home life is deteriorating further, and my mental health is too. Before Beacon House, I had to give up my bedroom and sanctuary for Janet's son. I am forced into sharing a room again with my little sister, who is four-and-a-half years my junior. I have never dealt well with sharing a room under normal circumstances, so the idea of sharing one when I am mentally unwell distresses me further.

I get angry because I am trying so hard, but no matter what I do, I can do nothing right. One day, I drive my brother to school, but when I get back Janet interrogates me. She corners me. She talks about how I don't want the house to change, but it's going to happen anyway and that it's her way or the highway. I don't like it when she talks to me like that. It is like she's trying to teach me a lesson or something. She's not my mother, and she's not my therapist. I want my dad to be happy, so I pretend to like her and go along with her and what is going on. I tell myself I don't like the changes because it is forcing me to accept the death of my mother and I'm not ready to do that yet. Again, reinforcing to myself that I am just being a bad child.

My family and I basically live parallel lives. We sleep under the same roof and occasionally eat together, but we do not talk. I cannot remember ever being asked how my day has been or how I am feeling today. We do not say good night or good morning. We exist together, but separate. Totally dysfunctional.

Until now, my dad has not taught me many life skills. I don't know how to properly clean a house or maintain a yard. I know how to vacuum (but not move furniture) and wash the floor. I don't know how to get rid of stuff I don't use anymore (our house would appear to be almost as bad as a low-grade hoarder). Outside, my brother cuts the lawn, but I don't think we even own a weed-eater. The garden is just weeds, our prized weed being the thistle that grows as high as the second-floor window. My father tries several times to kill it, but it just comes back. Eventually, he gives up on fighting it and we just let it grow. It is the ultimate symbol of resilience. We do rake the leaves, as we have three large trees on the property. I am also not introduced to a variety of foods, and I am such a picky eater that it's embarrassing to go over to other people's houses. My food comes from a box (yes, even mashed potatoes) unless it is homemade pizza or my grandmother cooks it.

My dad takes me to see my mother's grave (well—technically a wall). I have never been there since she died seven years ago. He has not had her plaque engraved despite all of these years. When I get home, Janet questions me about how I felt when I went to see my mom. She doesn't understand that this is not her place to ask and is making things worse. It turns out that my father told her how I reacted, completely shattering any trust I have in him. What I say and do while at my mom's grave is mine and my dad's business. Not hers.

I need to process everything that is going on, but no one gives me time or space to do so. They think I know how I feel and process everything immediately, but I don't. Now I can no longer talk to my dad about anything. He shares it all. Why can't they understand I don't want to be a prissy little spoiled kid, but that's all I know how to be? When she tells me it's her way or the highway, I don't know how to process that. What I get from that conversation is that whether or not I like it, changes are going to happen, so I'd better get on board. That, in reality, it doesn't matter if I like it, because my opinion doesn't matter (even though they want me to think it does.) That is so frustrating for me.

"My son gets up and faces the world despite his learning disability," Janet tells me one day.

I quickly realize I don't want to be compared to someone, especially her son. Why can't they understand I don't know how to process all of this?

When my dad gets home, I will be in trouble for this conversation. Being bitter is something I can't help myself from feeling. I mean, who wouldn't be? I've been on edge, unable to relax for more than a week. I have nowhere to go relax and 'process' all the information that's being put in my head.

It's no wonder my thoughts are all muddled up when I'm trying to think something through. I'm just so frustrated because I don't know how to react. I have no example to follow, and my logic is missing. So, what am I supposed to do? I know what I need to do. I need to get out of this situation, but I still don't have my own room. I can't relax in someone else's room. I want my dad to hire someone to finish the room in the basement, and I even offer to find a way to pay for it. However, it seems my sanity is not worth paying for someone to finish the room. So, I am stuck with my sister, my mind getting worse and worse and unable to process anything.

I don't know how to process it all, especially when she compares me to her son, as if I'm not trying. She doesn't get that I gave up MY room so they could move in, and pretended to be happy so that everything would be okay. I am trying SO DAMN HARD. There are conflicting messages I am receiving. I am told to say what I feel, but when I do, I get in trouble. I don't believe them anymore, and I don't trust what they say. So, I will not say anything.

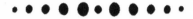

1997

When my mom got sick, my grandparents made a temporary move to Pickering to help. They rented a basement apartment from a neighbour because they needed to make such a quick move to help. The basement they rented was a few doors down the street and had two bedrooms (one of which was occupied by our neighbour's son), an eat-in kitchen, living room, and a full bathroom. When it became clear that she was gravely ill, they bought a house in our neighbourhood a few streets over. My mom and aunt purchased the house while my grandparents were on vacation. My mom and aunt picked it out, being able to see the 'good bones' in the layout. But the house was dirty, stank of smoke, had terrible carpets, and was very much neglected. My grandparents were on vacation, and when they returned, my mom and Aunt Tina had already purchased the house. My Gran told me many years later that she nearly cried when she saw the house because it was in such poor repair. However, once they had the floors redone, had the walls painted, and had new carpet put down, it was liveable. My grandparents continued to do renovations over the years, including installing a fireplace, which eventually becomes a source of comfort for me.

Monday, January 23rd, 2006

Amelia helps me prepare to talk with Janet about what is and is not helping me. Like trying to give me advice, insisting I share my feelings with her, and generally to stop trying to be my mother. In other words, I need her to leave me alone. I talk with Janet and things are better for a bit. I volunteer at the school again, and I am a lunchroom monitor for the special needs classes. This position is paid, which is helpful. It is too late to join the various teams and groups of cadets, thus I focus on keeping well. I might go back to Beacon house, so it's best not to join.

My mind is racing, and I can barely sleep. I continue to attend therapy with Amelia. However, our work turns away from processing my mother's death and focuses instead on surviving day-to-day life at home. I am convinced the key to my success is having a long-term therapist who will stick with me through my good and bad times. I have really internalized the message that my problems are all behavioural and I'm just a prissy little spoiled kid. Life at home is confusing and toxic. I continue to receive contradictory messages: we want you to take care of yourself and practice self-care, but only when it is convenient for us. We want you to learn to experience your emotions, let go, and cry, but if you do, we will punish you. With these mixed messages, my mental health keeps deteriorating further.

• • • ● ● • ● ● • • •

Saturday, January 28th, 2006

My weight is causing me distress. I have gained thirty pounds since my first hospital stay just three months ago. I want to get off the Zyprexa, as I know it is making me gain weight and slowing my metabolism. Zyprexa is what's known as an atypical antipsychotic, meaning it is a newer generation antipsychotic. Its role is to clarify what's going on in my mind. They typically use it for people with psychotic disorders like schizophrenia or mood disorders with psychotic features like severe mania or depression. It is known for working well but has severe metabolic effects, meaning people who take the medication typically gain lots of weight in a short amount of time. I don't know the psychiatrist's reasoning behind giving me this medication when I am being told I am not sick and told I am certainly not psychotic. I think it is being used as a chemical restraint because of some of the emotion-flattening side effects it has. Still, it is a powerful medication to put someone on when you don't believe they are actually psychotic.

I wish I had my own room, but I still do not. I am not sleeping well, but in my own room I could at least lie awake in peace. Instead, I listen to Danielle's snoring. Most nights I go to bed with multiple stuffed animals, not for comfort but to use as ammunition. I throw them at her when she snores too loud. It causes her to roll over and stop for a few minutes. I also do nothing at all. There is no room to work out. I can't surf the web from Danielle's room, and I hesitate to touch anything around the house for fear of getting into trouble. I get more and more stressed about my weight; I am fat and I can't live with myself in this state. In fact, all I seem to think about lately is food. Do I want to eat this? Should I eat that? Do I actually enjoy feeling hungry or is it just because I feel like that's when I'm losing the pounds? I don't know. I spent time today trying to do a Sudoku puzzle, but I should go out for a bike ride to lose some weight. I have been attending a dart group for a few years, perhaps tomorrow I will bike to the group.

Monday, January 30th, 2006

Today, Amelia and I are discussing how my father is not changing to meet my needs. We talk about how I can prompt him to ask me how my day was. I speak about my mom a bit, but I have a hard time showing emotion around that or anything to do with my mom, and we discuss this as well. One of these days, I will ask my dad what day she died and what day she was born. The psychiatrist agrees to wean me off the Zyprexa because of the weight gain. He does not raise the Zoloft, my antidepressant. I am going to see him again next week after my session with Amelia.

Wednesday, February 1st, 2006

I am working on finishing my room in the basement. I'm putting up metal plates to protect the wires and putting up insulation in the walls. I'm on less medication now, therefore I'm sleeping as well as can be expected. In other words, not well. I've been thinking a lot about Beacon House. I'm not sure that I want to go back. I want to get better, but I don't want to give up cadets and my friends. I'm struggling to decide.

Thursday, February 2nd, 2006

Today is the first day of the new semester in school. French, arts and crafts, and weight training are my classes this semester. I took French so I could graduate with my French bilingual certificate. I've completed twelve years of French schooling, and I'm not about to give up on it when I am one credit away.

I'm also stressed about cadets. Gordon, the lead cadet (Warrant Officer First Class) for our squadron, is being a real ass. There are certain things which are highly desired in cadets, such as getting to wear a lanyard or white belt. They are more formal and make us feel high class. Gordon is abusing his power by trying to make James give up his lanyard and yelling at us for getting white belts for the flag party.

This evening I am sad, so I am going to do as Amelia suggests. I write my feelings in my journal, then close the book to do something else. I'm not sure why I am so sad, but I suspect it has to do with going back to school where I have no friends.

I have been thinking about the "It was all for attention" thing. I don't think it was a "Look at me, look at me" but more so a "Something is wrong and I don't know how to communicate it". It was never a ploy to be childish.

They tell me I was crying for help, so I guess that's what it is.

Tuesday, February 7th, 2006

The drywall is going up in my room today. I am frustrated that it has taken this long. My dad and Janet announced their marriage in the summer, so why didn't they think ahead to where everyone would sleep? Or did they really think that taking away my room and giving it to her son was going to be totally okay and not distressing to me in the least? That I would just stay indefinitely in Danielle's room and be totally okay with it? Anyway, now that the drywall is up, Maggie is going to come help me paint. I am determined to eat almost nothing until I lose ten or fifteen pounds and look good again. When I can see my ribs, I will stop.

Wednesday, February 8th, 2006

Maggie comes to help me paint today. While we are looking for a paint roller, I have to decide whether to ask Janet if she knows where it is or not. I know Janet will treat me as if I am rubbing it in her face that she doesn't know where something is in the house. So, I decide to call my dad at work to ask. Unfortunately, as I can do no right, Janet yells at me for bothering my dad at work. At least this time I have a witness to the behaviour. A witness who does, in fact, verify the attitude I am receiving as not simply being in my head. In my friend's words, "What a bitch!"

Thursday, February 9th, 2006

I've been on this diet for a few days now and it's the greatest idea I've ever had. I'm burning calories all day, sleeping well at night, and losing pounds. I feel great, and I'm going to look great too. It won't be long, as I'm down to 145-146 pounds.

I have to decide if I'm going to talk to Amelia about my weird, bad thoughts. Like why I want to starve myself and why I wish bad things happened to me? Not passing school and never amounting to anything is another bad thought for me. I don't want to be poor, but I don't know if I have the smarts to amount to anything. I can't memorize anything. I'll never make it at university. I thought I wanted to do nursing, but now I don't know if I can handle nursing school. I had also thought about Occupational Therapy, but even OTA (OT Assistant) school is a lot of work that my brain cannot handle. Would I even get paid well enough as an OTA to live well? I want to have a good quality of life if I'm going to be alive.

Many people have not heard of Occupational Therapy unless they have been in a situation to need an Occupational Therapist. Occupational Therapy looks at the activities that *occupy* someone's time; dressing, bathing, toileting, meal preparation, mobility, sleep, and more. An OT assistant is someone who works in OT but does not have the full qualifications of an OT. In Ontario, it is a two-year college diploma to become an Occupational Therapist Assistant/Physical Therapist Assistant.

Journal Entry: Friday, February 10th, 2006
I know there will be a confrontation tonight at dinner. But I will hold strong. I will refuse to eat the contaminated food

and water. The government is controlling our minds with the pesticides they put in our foods. They spray them on the crops. I have enough fat on my body to survive until I can think of a solution. It's those Americans; they are controlling us so we don't turn against them. So that we support them.

Journal Entry: Saturday, February 11th, 2006

I've figured it out. It's not the government adding mind-control agents to our foods. It's stuff that gives you cancer so that the drug companies can test new drugs on you. My mom is talking to me about the food and water that is giving her cancer.

I go to her grave/ wall. I only have twenty dollars, so I take a cab as far as he will take me, then I walk the rest of the way. I don't care that it is nighttime or cold out.

There is a bench outside my mom's wall. I sit on it for a while until the security guard finds me. He brings me home, but my dad and Janet are not home.

Gosh, I don't know what I'm going to do. It's like my mind has a mind of its own. One moment I hear Mom talking to me, then I'm waiting in the hospital, and the next I'm being ordered around by Janet. I hate my mind. Something is wrong and I can't figure out what. I don't know what's bothering me. Is it because I feel like Dad doesn't love me anymore or is it I feel like he doesn't love Mom anymore? I mean, what the hell is going on with my mind? I have myself so convinced that I hear Mom. I don't know if I really hear her or if I'm just making myself believe I do. I just don't know.

And why do I suddenly feel this way again? I mean, I want to go to college and be something, right? So how come I keep putting off applying, and why do I keep sabotaging myself? I mean, why am I so impulsive? It's like I think something and then I automatically have to act on it and I don't have the sense in me or the capability to snap out of it. I'm so worried that Amelia is going to give up on me, too. Right now, she's the only person I have. The only one. My dad doesn't understand, and even if I want to talk to him, all our conversations have to include Janet now. I don't know how I'm going to survive. Right now I'd love to throw myself off a bridge, but I keep remembering what a teacher at school said: that if I die, there will be a lot of sad people and many people who will miss me. But really, what if Amelia gives up on me, too? My dad has already given up on me and I'm scared to tell my friends anything because I don't want them to give up on me too. I suggested going back to Beacon House, and my dad didn't think that's what I needed. But I do. I really think I have a problem with my personality. I mean, why else would I do the things I do? I just don't understand myself. I wish I did.

I'm still really confused about this whole Mom thing. Did I really hear her voice or was that just a voice in my mind? And was it while I was there at her wall (because everything was such a blur) or did I dream it maybe? I don't know. I mean, the last time I was hearing voices and stuff, it was just my mind playing tricks on me. And once I figured out how to control it, I could. At least, I can while I am taking medication. But how come this time I can't? Why am I so convinced that eating will give me cancer and that my mom spoke to me? I just don't understand. Is it real? Are these thoughts real? Or is my mind playing games with itself? I just don't know.

I keep thinking back to the days at Beacon House and the worker asking me, "What do I get out of all of this?" I mean, it makes no sense! All that happens is my dad gets mad at me and I end up hurting myself. So why do I keep doing it? Am I really doing it? Is it actually under my control? I just don't understand. I don't believe that this has anything to do with my mom, right? I mean, it doesn't connect. Sabotaging myself, my mind, just doesn't make sense. I wish I could make myself right. I mean, I try, and it works for a little while, and then I sabotage my progress. Am I scared of getting well? And if so, why? What am I scared of?

I am thinking of moving out. I don't understand why I can't adapt to these changes like everyone else. Why am I fighting this so much? Shouldn't I be happy for my dad for being happy? Or am I mad at myself for not being able to make my dad happy enough? Or am I mad at him for trying to replace Mom? Gosh, my mind is such a mess right now. Just a mess. It's all muddled, full of things I don't understand, and I'm so scared that something will happen again. What if it does and I really get kicked out of the house? Janet keeps telling me it's her way or the highway and I want so badly to take the highway. And I don't understand why I want to, because I know that if I do, I'll lose contact with my family and I'll end up living on the streets until I die if I don't kill myself first. Gosh, am I ever screwed up!

I am brought, again, by my father to the hospital and left there, but I am not admitted. He doesn't know how

to deal with my nonsensical thinking. Things are such a
blur. I don't remember much at all.

Journal Entry: Tuesday, February 14th, 2006.

*I fear the water calling me again. What if I lose it and my
dad just kicks me out? What if he doesn't bother to take me to
the hospital? Or what if they don't realize that I can't 'snap
out of it'? I'm so afraid I'll end up living on the street, not
understanding what's going on. I'm not sure I can control it
forever.*

*I think Dad and Janet had a fight and now my dad's mad
at me again. They keep getting mad at me. Mad at me for
things I don't even realize I am doing wrong. Like with the
TV last night. I was only doing what was normal for me, to
watch what I wanted. I never knew it was 'disrespectful' to not
ask everyone in the room if it was okay. How was I supposed
to know? My family has never done this. It's always been first
come, first served. And even when I do this, I am met with a
"see I had to teach her that" response and attitude from Janet.*

*My best course of action is to no longer talk unless spoken
to. I just get in trouble for saying the wrong things. Stories I
think are funny are just upsetting to other people and then I
get in trouble. I'm just not going to do it anymore. I will not
be bad. I'm always trying to be good, but I'm just not good
enough. Not good enough to do things right, not good enough
to make people happy. Maybe I would just be better off in
my own little world. Then I could hurt no one. Maybe I'd
be better off dead. It'd hurt them at first, but they all seem
capable of getting over deaths just fine.*

The only one who seems to care even remotely is my brother, who came with me to the hospital last Saturday. He couldn't stay and I sat there alone for hours. They didn't admit me. I think if things get worse, I'm going to throw myself off a bridge, maybe onto highway 401. Then I can leave behind all the people that hate me.

Journal Entry: Thursday, February 16th, 2006

Today I had an appointment with Amelia. I told her about what has happened at home and the hospital, and she helped me sort through it. She tried to make me realize I am not a bad kid, but I know I am. She wants me to bring my dad with me next week if we are still having problems.

Chapter 7

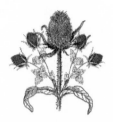

J ournal Entry: Monday, February 20th, 2006

Finally, this weekend we finished my room—six months after they announced their engagement and two months after they got married, subsequently kicking me out of my room. I finally have a place of my own.

I am getting so annoyed with Janet. I don't like that she keeps trying to parent me. She's trying to parent me over my dad, and my dad's just letting her. She keeps getting on me to find a job; she's mentioned it three times so far today. I have told her already that I am looking and she doesn't need to keep nagging me so much.

I noticed Danielle got annoyed with her on Sunday, too. Jennifer (home from university), Danielle, and I were trying to get the wardrobe down the stairs. Janet was just watching, of course, and not actually helping. Jennifer joked that all of our effort was just going to result in my dad coming up and helping anyway, and sure enough, when he did, Janet said, "If you guys hadn't been so loud..." like it was all our fault that we aren't strong enough and my dad had to help. So, Danielle got mad. Later at Gran's for dinner, I asked if Dad thought we might be able to put the door on tonight. Janet rolled her eyes, like "how dare I ask such a thing". She's a nice lady and all, but a bitch to live with.

Even today, when Brian and I were talking about shelves, she made this face when I told her that my dad had said to use different brackets. And when I was talking about maybe rearranging my room, she came in and gave another suggestion, and when I told her I didn't enjoy having my bed in the middle of the room, she kept pushing it.

I swear, she treats me like I'm the reason her world is not perfect. She makes me feel like everything is my fault. And I hate how she has my dad wrapped around her finger. But on the plus side, now I have my room, where I can go to stay away from her. Gosh, she is so controlling!

Journal Entry: Wednesday, February 22nd, 2006

I have lost all hope. My dad has given up on me. I'm going to get cancer, and there's nothing I can do about it. I'm so lonely. The only person I thought I could count on has deserted me. I feel so worthless. I'm a bad person. I never thought I was, but I must be. Why else would my dad no longer care? I know the world would be better off without me. If only I hadn't said what they wanted to hear, that it was all for attention. Even now, I don't know why the 'dissociating' was happening, but I knew I had to control it. I also knew that they wouldn't let me out to go to the wedding, so I made up a reason it was happening. And now my dad thinks it's all an act. To get his attention. Well, you know what? I don't want his attention, or his sympathy. I want his support. I want to come home from a bad day and talk about it with him. Cry if I need to. Not come home and try to be forced into talking by Janet. Or to open up and have Janet take away more of my privileges (like being allowed to have a door to cry in private in my room). I want support. But my dad has given up. I have nothing left. Now I'm under so much stress again that I'm scared the dissociations will start again. I just don't know how to handle all this. I don't think I can do it anymore.

I can't deal with her trying to force me to talk. Or him giving up on me. My world makes no sense. If I cry, she threatens to take away my door if I don't share my innermost feelings with her. But when I do share, I am told that I am exaggerating, making things up, doing this for attention.

One day, she came down to my room, totally unprovoked, and told me her therapist told her to tell me she hates me. I'm not sure how that was supposed to help the situation at all.

I'm ready to quit. I really am. I'm sick of all this. I'm a horrible person. I don't deserve to live. Horrible, horrible person. I don't deserve to live. I deserve to be beaten and whipped. And killed. I don't deserve to be alive.

Journal Entry: Thursday, February 23rd, 2006

I am so scared. What if my dad kicks me out? What am I going to do? I'm such a bad person. My dad has given up on me. I have no one but my friends, but I can't put this on them either. It's not fair and that would make me an even more horrible person. I don't understand why I'm so bad. What am I doing wrong? I want to cry into my dad's shoulder, but he has given up on me. If he kicks me out, there is no point in going on. What am I going to do? I'm so afraid. I'm going to lie on the train tracks and kill myself. None of these pills or cutting shit. I deserve to die. I'm worthless. I don't know how to convince my dad not to give up on me, but the reality is he already has. I must really be a horrible person.

I'm beyond saving. I deserve to be beaten. I deserve to be slashed. I just wish I could hurt myself. I deserve it. But if I do, then I get kicked out. I'm afraid to talk to my dad about all of this. What if he kicks me out? I'm only trying to make things better. I can't deal with him kicking me out. He's already said that he wants to. How can I stop him? I can't. I must really be a horrible person if he wants to get rid of me. I don't deserve to be alive. Sure, I do good things, but what's the point? All the help in the world won't make things better. I'm so afraid that he's going to kick me out. I can't survive that.

Journal Entry: Friday, February 24th, 2006

Yesterday I had my meeting with Amelia. My dad came in and we talked about what has been going on at home. Amelia got him to make a deal that he would ask Janet to leave me alone and I would take care of myself (eating, not always in my room). So far, things are better, and my dad gave permission to have some friends sleep over to celebrate my new room.

Journal Entry: Thursday, March 2nd, 2006

Sometimes I can't decide. One day I'm ready to move on, do something productive with my life, and then 2 minutes later I'm so depressed that I'm ready to no longer exist. I don't feel like I'm worth something, anything. I'm a worthless piece of crap that's never going to accomplish anything. It's so frustrating. Up, down, up, down. I never know how I'm going to feel in a couple of minutes.

Yesterday was 3 months of no cutting. I am happy about this and told a teacher and 2 friends. I don't dare tell Dad or Janet; I need someone to be happy with me and not get on me about having started doing it in the first place. But sometimes I just want to become nothing. No longer exist. Be taken away to a mental hospital and locked up. I just don't know how to deal with my problems. I just want to become nothing again. Like I was those 6 weeks in the hospital. I wish I hadn't told them what they wanted to hear to get out. I wish I hadn't told them it was all to get my dad's attention.

I'm tired of fighting. What would happen if I killed myself? What if I stopped fighting it and let the wanderings happen? I'm so afraid that the monsters are going to come after me again, then I know I'll lose control. Right now, my mom says they don't know where I am. She's the one who lets me know when they are after me. I'm scared all the time now. It's only a matter of time before they get here. Do I tell Amelia this? How do I know she's not in on it with them? How do I know?

Journal Entry: March 6th, 2006

I can't think straight today. The walls are breathing. I can't concentrate when I'm driving. I went 160 km/hr by accident on the 401. It's a good thing I didn't get into an accident. I have zero attention span and I can't pay attention in class.

March 14th, 2006

It is March break, and I'm working at camp during the day. I am tired after a long day working at the camp and decide to practice my self-care. My therapist, my dad, and even Janet have told me I need to learn to take care of myself. So, today I plan my evening, to have a bath and go to bed early. No one tells me they will pack up Janet's house tonight.

So, when the phone rings at 8:30 p.m. and I hear my younger sister saying, "Come help us pack and move Janet's stuff," I stand up for myself.

"No, I'm not coming, as I have planned to go to bed at 9:00 p.m. I'm taking care of myself tonight."

A few minutes later, I get another call, this time from Janet.

"Get your lazy ass down here and start helping!" she yells.

It is already dark out. I am ready for bed. So, grudgingly, I get out of bed and drive to the next town over to where her home is located. We, the Grace kids, have to help pack her house. Her children are not there.

"It's all your father's fault," Janet rants, focusing her comments toward me.

"How is this Liz's fault?" my little sister Danielle asks.

"You want to sit with your dad?" Janet states in a matter-of-fact way (referring to when I tried to sit next to him on the couch a night or two ago). "Well, I am NOT going to let you!"

In the end, I help pack until I am given permission to go home, feeling shitty about myself and even more depressed. I go to bed and wake up extra exhausted in the morning.

Journal Entry: March 15ᵗʰ, 2006

Janet and Dad are constantly giving me conflicting information. First, they say to put myself first, but when I do, Janet says it doesn't matter what I want/need. It's so confusing, I don't understand.

- *Things she has said to me I can think of right now:*

- *She hates me*

- *She is going to take her son and leave*

- *I MUST use the shower downstairs and am not permitted to shower in the tub/shower upstairs, even though I hate the downstairs shower*

- *That I manipulate my therapist and I should get a new therapist*

- *That she and my dad spent a lot of time and money building my room, so how dare I keep it such a mess*

- *I'm immature because I still drink milk out of the cereal bowl*

- *I thump around the house*

- *I cause most/almost all the problems*

- *She understands that I'm dealing with issues with my mother, but that I'd better get over it quick*

I think it's horrible that her desire to hurt me is stronger than her desire to love my father. She would rather walk out on him to hurt us both. On Thursday, I'm going to ask my dad to come to see Amelia with me. And I want to hear from him what is going on. I will not tell him the shit that she's told me. I want to hear it from him, and I want to know if he gave her permission to give me these little "talks".

Journal Entry April 1, 2006

Last night, I had a great time throwing a surprise eighteenth birthday party for Kathy. We even blew up condom balloons. I actually enjoyed it. This morning I went for a tour of Humber College. I really liked the campus and wanted to go there. I actually feel a bit more motivated to work for my high school diploma.

April 1 , 2006

When I get home from touring Humber College, I talk about colleges with Dad and Janet. This leads to a huge fight when Janet immediately, snidely, comments, "How can you know if you have only been to one school?"

I leave the house to let off some steam at dragon boat practice, then I go to a friend's house to figure out what I'm going to do. I realize I can't do this anymore.

Chapter 8

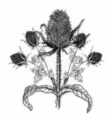

A PRIL 3RD, 2006

  I don't know what to do anymore. I need to get out of the house. I'm the problem. If it wasn't for me, then everyone would be happy. I can't move away, because that would make me more unhappy. Sure, I wouldn't be at home, but I wouldn't be able to do the stuff I like to do any more like sports, cadets, and my friends. I might have to quit high school.

<u>Moving Out</u>
Option A

- *Get full time job*

- *Quit school*

- *No activities*

Option B
- *Find someone to live with*

- *Get job to help pay rent*

- *No college*

- *Get full time job once done with high school*

- *No activities*

First week of April 2006
When I talk to Amelia, she encourages me to find someplace else to stay. With that encouragement, I talk with my grandparents, who offer me the guest bedroom. I don't accept when we talk, but I want to know what my options are.

A few days later, I have the flu and feel terrible. I stay home from school and stay in bed, wrapped tight in my covers. I get a knock at my bedroom door and it's one of Janet's daughters,

"Are you attending the family meeting tonight?"

"No one told me about it." I say, "I am sick, but I guess I can be there".

That evening, the so-called 'family meeting' turns out to be a 'shit on Liz meeting' where I am blamed for every wrong in both the household and with Janet's mental health. I'm fed up and I've had enough of it.

"I have already spoken to my grandparents," I say, "Who have offered for me to stay there if I want."

After that, I storm back down to my room and curl back up into my covers.

Not even twenty-four hours later, my father takes me in his van to talk after getting me hot chocolate and himself a coffee from Tim Hortons. We park by the water.

"I think it's best if you move in with your grandparents. You will always be welcome at home … it will be more like you have two homes." He took a couple of sips of his coffee. "You should get a job and pay them rent."

Journal Entry: April 10th, 2006

Yesterday, I moved in with my grandparents. I will have two homes but most of my time will be with my grandparents, as things are not going well at my father's home. I have been tossing and turning for two weeks, and the past two nights I barely slept at all.

April 16th, 2006

Gran and Grandad have gone away for a week to Boston to visit my Aunt Tina. It is a long weekend (Easter), and my friend Maggie is home from university. Friday night we go to a party at a friend's house, and although we bring alcohol, I don't even finish one cooler. I'm too scared to lose control. For the same reason, I don't try any of the marijuana going around (not to mention I hate the smell of it).

Saturday, I have plans to help Danielle and Brian make pizza, but when I get there, they have already made it. Danielle and I rent a movie to watch, and my brother Brian gets home around 9:00 p.m. Danielle doesn't want to come back with me to Gran's. There is nowhere for me to sleep at my dad's house, so I return to my grandparent's house.

Later during the weekend, there is an argument between Janet, myself, and my father. I'm not sure about what. Maybe he and Janet want me to do something? I'm not sure. I only remember parts of what happens next. I'm not sure why they come over. Are they angry about something I've said? Are they concerned? I know they come into the house, and I am talking about getting the fog out of my blood. I have a razor and am trying to cut it out. They call an ambulance, who call the cops, who try to handcuff me on the floor. I am combative, trying to get away while they rush me to the hospital where they again restrain me physically and chemically.

At the hospital, I am surrounded by security, and a nurse gives me a shot of something. I fight as hard as I can.

"I thought you said this stuff would work immediately," I hear one of the guards say, before I pass out asleep.

I am vaguely aware of being pushed in a wheelchair, then undressed in a bathroom. I wake up in the Psychiatric Intensive Care Unit (PICU), strapped to a bed. My wrists and ankles are bound with baby blue cuffs. I don't understand why they are restraining me. I was asleep, and now, I'm calm. I try everything I can think of to get the staff to let me out. Eventually, they let me go to the bathroom, but then, despite being calm, put me back in restraints. Like a punishment. Or maybe they actually believe the load of BS about restraints being calming and reassuring to the patient (hint: they are not).[1]

"Please, please don't put me back in those restraints. Please. I promise to be good. Please don't. Don't put those back on me. Please!" I beg.

But the nurse doesn't care.

"Either you let me do it or I will call security to do it," she says, through clenched teeth.

"What is going on?" the psychiatrist asks while seated in the interview room.

"I have this fogginess in my blood and that I need to get it out," I tell him.

"How did it get there?" he inquires.

"The government."

When I am feeling a bit better, on April 19th, 2006, my father comes to visit. He sits with me in a quiet room.

"You are no longer welcome at home," he tells me flat out. Just one sentence, then he walks out.

Yet again, I have nowhere to go. Thanks to mental illness, my father wants nothing to do with me. I can't imagine if I had a brain tumour that he would treat me this way and kick me out of the house for behaviour he does not understand. I do not know if my grandparents will allow me back into their home. Maybe this world will be better without me. I can't seem to control this. I call my grandfather.

"When can I pick you up?" he asks without hesitation.

At eighteen, this is my first memorable experience of unconditional love.

Chapter 9

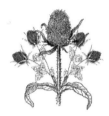

April 20th, 2006

My father has officially deserted me. I am no longer welcome at home. His exact words. I hate that my father can't see that I have a mental illness. I'm not just making this up. It's not 'behaviour'. He is not a man of his word. Just last week, he told me I would always have that house as a home. He has changed.

April 24th, 2006

I should have moved ages ago. Returning to my grandparents' home means a return to stability and unconditional love. Something, up to this point, I've had no concept of. I am broken, but my grandparents get me up every day, make sure I wear clean clothes and eat breakfast. My grandmother makes me lunch, as I am in no shape to do so myself. She makes dinner every night,

sometimes two different dishes, in order to make sure
there is something I will eat. A few times a week, they
insist I shower. Every single day, they drive me to and
pick me up from school. They also drive me to therapy
appointments until I am eventually well enough to drive
myself. They literally nurse me back to health. I'm sure it
is very difficult for them to see their granddaughter like
this, and I will always credit them with my recovery and
survival.

School consists of French, weight training, and arts
and crafts. I need the credits and the French class to
graduate, and so that is what I focus on. And yes, weight
training and arts and crafts really are worth high school
credits and in their own regard are therapy. Exercise and
creativity. French is the hardest subject, as there is actual
homework to be completed. I mostly do this in my 'spare'
or free period.

I continue to volunteer with the special education classes at my high school. One student was off school last
year and has totally lost his life skills. He cannot feed
himself, but I work with him every day to help him
learn to regain that skill. At first, I do hand over hand
with him, slowly reducing the amount of support I give.
By the end of the year, he is feeding himself, even if
slowly. This solidifies for me my decision to become
an Occupational Therapist Assistant and provides more
motivation to graduate.

My marks aren't great, but I pass by enough to be accepted to college in the fall. My grandparents encourage
me and tell me I have no limits. I visited another school

a while ago, but it just confirms my original thought;
Humber is right for me.

Summer 2006

Over the summer, my health continues to improve. I
stop seeing Amelia, as I am working as a camp counsellor
at a day camp and cannot take the time off.

I am also part of an elite dragon boat team. Dragon
boat racing is a competition between boats that consist
of twenty paddlers, a coxswain, and a drummer. The
paddlers are seated in pairs for ten rows of paddlers in
each boat. For the past two years, we have been working
toward competing at the Club Crew World Championships (CCWC) in Toronto, summer 2006. I find I am
constantly asking my seat partner to repeat the instructions, as I cannot hear what the coach is saying.

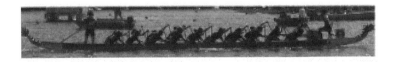

I am also playing soccer in a women's intercity league.
I can drive myself and it gets me out of the house another
night of the week. I play goalie, so there is not as much
exercise, but my confidence slowly increases. One night,
the field is really muddy, as it has been raining. During
the game, I dive for several balls, resulting in me being

covered in mud. When the game finishes, I am left trying to decide how to get home without ruining the car. I rig up a series of plastic bags and a towel so that I can get home without getting mud on the seat. When I get home, I have another problem; how do I get up to the shower without dripping mud everywhere?

"Gran!" I say as I open the door a crack. "Can you bring me a big towel?"

She does, sees the mud and smiles.

"Thank you."

I strip off my muddy shorts, socks, shoes, and t-shirt right on the front porch, using the swimming pool changeroom technique of keeping a towel wrapped around myself while pulling off my clothes. In my bra and underwear, covered with a towel, I head up to the bathroom for a long shower, trying to get the water to run clear. We will laugh about this situation for years to come.

I find sports to be very therapeutic, producing endorphins from both the exercise and the socialization. The dragon boat team is on the water two-to-three times a week with dry-land training in addition. I usually play soccer once a week. I am losing a bit of the weight from the medications and becoming much stronger.

The summer wraps up and we enter the weekend of the World Club Crew Dragon Boat Championships. My grandparents want to come see me, and they take a taxi (an adventure of its own) to the park where it is being hosted. They watch from the bleachers as I compete, probably relieved at the change in my mental health from six months prior.

In June, my grandparents and I go see my sister's play in a small theatre in Pickering. We are sitting in the little waiting room, as the theatre is not yet open for us to go in. I am reading a magazine when suddenly my father comes up to us.

"Where do you get off?" he is loud, and he is making quite a scene, "Ignoring Janet like that?"

"Gran and Liz have been reading, and I nodded to Janet in acknowledgment when she came in," my grandfather calmly responds.

Apparently, this was not enough for her, and Janet threatened to leave my dad, end the marriage, and go home. Regardless, we go into the theatre and watch my sister's play. I assume they get their act together, come in, and sit calmly, but I'm not sure.

A few weeks later I am watching my sister's soccer game when I meet up (as pre-arranged) with my dad. We are chatting and he tells me he is happy. I note how he is happy *without me* being around. However, as we chat, suddenly Janet appears and hands him her rings.

"I am fed up and going away!" Janet and my father argue before she leaves.

He says nothing to me after that at the game, and I'm not sure how I am responsible for this fight, but they are certainly blaming me. My grandparents write a brief letter (that I am not privy to) stating their side of what happened when Janet accused them of being unfriendly toward her. My father does not reply.

All summer long, I prepare to go away to college. It is about one-and-a-half hours by transit, and it is planned that I will come home often during the school year. We rent a minivan, pack it with my stuff, and drive across the city on move-in day.

Part Two

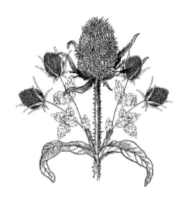

Chapter 10

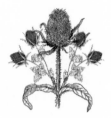

E ARLY 1990s

At some point when I was young, my mom took me for a hearing test, as I was always yelling. I must have been young, as I remember playing with blocks and being told to stack them when I heard the sound. I got distracted, and I just played with the blocks.

"Don't worry about it. She's just yelling because she's competing with her siblings," the audiologist told my mom.

As a teenager, I knew something was off, but I couldn't quite name what it was. When I was sixteen, I was working as a camp counsellor at a summer day camp. The other staff and I were eating lunch around a table in a big room. The kids had not yet come back from another portion of the camp. I remember looking around the table and realizing what was off. I couldn't understand what the other staff across the table were saying. There was not enough volume nor clarity for me to hear and decipher the conversation properly. It was comparable to when I received my first pair of glasses. The world had looked normal to me until I donned my glasses for the first time and realized there were things I could not see. Things that, previously, were absent from my vision, that now I was able to see. With the hearing loss, it wasn't a sudden thing; like one minute I could hear and the next I couldn't. It was more of an understanding of what was happening and why I was struggling. A 'light bulb' sort of moment. However, being a teenager, naturally I said nothing. I shrugged it off. I didn't want to be different from the other students, especially after my experiences with bullying. I worked harder to pay attention and didn't think about it again for a while.

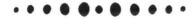

September 2006

Jumping into college is like starting over. I have a new group of people, a new group of expectations and a new set of responsibilities. I try to forget what happened during my final year of high school. I must put it behind me and focus on the future if I want to succeed. I use the strategies of burying and suppressing my emotions and experiences. This reinforces everything the hospital stays taught me, that I need to pretend as though I am like everyone else. I avoid telling anyone about my experiences with mental health. My bad experiences have left me ashamed, as though I am somehow at fault. I focus on the problem here and now—the problem of hearing in class and maintaining my improved mental health.

The public colleges in Ontario have disability departments to help students with disabilities succeed. I register, anticipating needing help with my mental health and soon realize that I need help with my hearing struggles as well. I request a diagnosis from my psychiatrist in Pickering to give to the Disability Services department at Humber. He writes a letter stating that I have 'adjustment disorder, abnormal grief, and histrionic personality traits'. Even after everything my social worker witnessed, my psychiatrist still thinks I was doing things for attention.

When classes start, I realize that college is not at all like high school. I actually want to learn but soon notice I cannot hear the speaker, even though, I am sitting in the front row. This leads to me getting a hearing test, where I am diagnosed with a mild hearing loss. The first set of hearing aids I get are red, but I still am experiencing difficulty hearing the lecturer. Disability Services recommends I receive an Assistive Listening Device[2], (ALD) which requires a distinct style of hearing aid. I get my hearing aids switched to a different model that only comes in boring brown. After that, it is a matter of finding funding for the device.

I have a small RESP[3], and therefore do not apply for the Ontario Student Assistance Program (OSAP)[4] this year. This makes finding funding difficult, as funding for disability equipment ties into getting funds from that program. When I ask my father for his and Janet's income information so I can apply for OSAP, I am told no. I write a letter explaining the situation, as do my grandparents, who have cared for me since they took me in, being hopeful that this would help me with the funding process. Nevertheless, OSAP declines my application. Eventually, the SDS[5] finds a donor who funds the device for me, as, without my father and Janet's income information, no one will consider my application.

Fall 2006

Throughout this time, I learn that living with hearing loss is not simply 'not hearing'. There is a lot of planning that goes into everything and an element of grief that I must overcome. One cannot just show up and expect to be accommodated. If I want to go to the movies, I have to check the listings for the showing with closed captions, book my tickets, and arrive early so I can get the closed captioning device (as the staff are never quite sure where they are). When they finally find a working one, I have to find a spot in the theatre where I can see both the captioning device and the screen.

Now that I can hear properly, I flourish. Suddenly I am somewhere I want to be. I have freedom and independence. I am responsible for getting myself to class, doing my homework, and studying for tests. In class, I am getting 90s and finding the material quite easy and interesting. My mood is higher than it has been in over a year.

Hanging out with friends when I have hearing loss is difficult. I can't control the background noise. Lip reading is difficult with poor lighting, when one is eating and when people do not know to face me when speaking to me. Other obstacles for the hard of hearing, include feeling left out of conversations, missing vital information and the lack of understanding by some individuals about how to address and accommodate those with a hearing loss. As well, patience needs to be exercised with those who have a hearing loss as they may need a longer time to process information. Often, hard-of-hearing people are left out of friend circles, unintentionally, because no one thinks to tell us that the group is meeting, or our difficulty communicating in a group leaves us as outsiders as others pair off. Or to do a group project where no one knows anything about my need to see faces, to wait for me to catch up, and to give me time to process is challenging.

During my first semester in residence, I fall in love with my independence. I live in a low rise building in a single room right next to the elevator. The room is small, just big enough for a single bed, mini fridge, desk, and closet. But it is my space to do what I want and have to share it with no one. I have a good number of friends, including one who I eye as a potential partner (nothing ever comes of it).

Residence has its downsides too. As a picky eater, I have a hard time finding food I will eat, often eating the same thing for days in a row. When I left for college, I ate a total of six vegetables (white potatoes, corn, peas, raw carrots, raw broccoli, and lettuce). As kids, we had mostly eaten pre-made, frozen foods, grilled cheese, and pizza. The only home-cooked meals we had were at my grandparents' house and occasionally some Beefaroni and Kraft Dinner (if you can consider these to be 'homemade'). When I moved in with my grandparents, I was hardly in a state where expanding my palette was a priority. I am embarrassed that I don't eat more foods and decide I want to work towards trying various new foods.

Spring 2007

School is another example of where hearing loss has an unexpected impact. While I am using an FM system at school, I have to show up early to class so that I have time to hand the speaker the mic and explain its use. Sometimes I have to convince the lecturer I am not recording anything, then find a seat near the front (but not the first row, I'm not *that* eager) where I can watch their face. At least once a day a professor will forget to turn the mic on, so I will have to raise my hand and wait for them to see me, stop talking (assuming I have a question), then finally turn it on. But profs never go back to the start of their lecture, so I often miss the intro for the lesson. One time, I didn't hear that there would be a quiz at the end of class and nearly missed the quiz. I only found out when I started to get up to pack my books and no one else did!

In my second semester of college, I apply to be a Resident Assistant. My sister inspired me as she was an RA at her university. I apply and am offered the job. It is difficult joining a team mid-year as training was at the beginning of the semester and the RA team is already established. They have gone away for training in the summer and worked together for an entire semester. Josh (the other new RA) and I are the odd people out. We support each other, and I enjoy running programs. But I have never been a popular kid, so it is difficult to get the floor involved when they have already established their (non)-community for a semester.

February 2007

I am at my grandparents' house and all is quiet, when suddenly there is a loud noise at the door. Janet and my father are there, yelling stuff and waving around a piece of paper.

"My daughter works for the police department! And she had them analyze this letter! And they said it was written by an eighteen-year-old French immersion girl!" Janet yells.

"*I* wrote that letter," my grandfather, who always remains calm, says to her coldly. "It is *my* signature on it, and Liz knows nothing about it."

It's true, I do not know what is going on.

I will learn later that my grandparents sent a letter to my dad and Janet about how they didn't like how my father had treated them despite them still treating him like a son. They hoped he didn't treat his own parents that way; how he behaved poorly at the theatre and to them in general. They wanted their key returned; they noted the grandkids were always welcome, but they wanted nothing more to do with him and Janet.

"We want to talk to Liz," my dad and Janet demand.

I think it over for a minute, and decide I will talk to them in public, where I assume she will not make a scene. So we go to Tim Hortons and talk again. Only this time, when the conversation moves away from what she wants, Janet takes off her rings, puts them on the table, and walks out. She is forcing my father to choose between his daughter and his wife. I, on the other hand, as enraged as I am, have no intention of making him choose, so I leave. He can go after her.

I am told this is not the last time she does this over the years, but I do not witness it again, as a little while after getting home from this mishap, I call my father. I am frustrated.

"I am done being the one to try in this relationship. The ball is now in your court." I tell him, "If you want to continue to have a relationship with me, your daughter, then it is up to you to make that happen. I'm done."

I never hear from him again.

There is a bit of friction with one of the two Residence Life Coordinators. I make some mistakes, as you would expect of a new hire in the middle of the year, one of which concerns a meeting with the Senior RA. Josh, the other new RA and I are to meet the senior RA in the RA room, but when we get there, she is doing something else. She never joins us, so we aren't sure what to do. I am sure that I left at the right time, and I remember checking the clock. But the Coordinator and the Senior RA tell me I was late and try to make it sound like I am lying about what time I showed up. I am very clear with them. I did not lie about what time I thought I got there. Is it possible I read the clock wrong? Sure. But I did not knowingly lie about the time. However, that seems to leave them with a chip on their shoulders. I think Josh has his own unpleasant experiences, as we are both feeling like the outsiders on the residence team.

As I am taking over a position for an RA who left, I do not have an official RA vest. First, I borrow one of the other staff's vests when it is my turn to be on call. Eventually, they find me a vest from the staff member who left. I go to my RLC's office, but she is not there, although I can see the vest in her office. The other RLC, who is in her office, offers to get it for me. I don't know why not; thus, she gets it and gives it to me. Later, I see my RLC and she is surprised to see me with the vest. Her jaw drops as if I went into her office and took it. Obviously, I could not have done so as she had locked the door! Even if it was open, I would never have removed something from someone's office! However, it seems to give her yet another reason to dislike me.

When selection for next year's staff team happens, I find myself in an impossible situation. I feel like they have set me up to fail. The interview is a group interview where they ask us, a group of RAs, to plan the RA orientation training with a student who has low vision. The problem is, I never attended the initial training, I have not experienced the orientation. How am I supposed to contribute to something I have not experienced when everyone else in the room has? Needless to say, I bomb the interview and am not rehired. Looking back, I wonder if I should have provided my experience toward including the RA with vision loss. On the other hand, how was I supposed to relate my mild hearing loss to that, or is it even a reasonable expectation for me to have to go so far out of my comfort zone to contribute something to the group compared to what they expect of the other returning staff members?

During the second semester, I get depressed again. I feel sad and alone, tired and unmotivated. I find it hard to relate to people and concentrate. I push through, and throughout the semester and into the summer, I return home to my grandparents' home.

Summer 2007

The second summer living with my grandparents I work at camp again. I also start a collection of carnivorous plants. It starts with one Venus fly trap I purchase at a local store, then I order a few more online. I get several varieties over the summer, and it gives me something to keep me busy. I'm responsible for feeding (literally) and watering the plants. My grandparents are very patient with me taking care of these plants and setting up a mini greenhouse on the deck. I suspect they are relieved to see me showing interest in something that has a longer-term commitment.

September 2007

In my second year of college, I share a two-bedroom suite with a suite-mate, Jane. She is friendly and I learn a lot about how other families function. The humour that I grew up with turns out to not be humorous to most other people. I have grown up with a 'put down' style of humour, where you make fun of the other person or make them feel bad for fun. I learn that is not the norm when I am joking with my suite-mate and say something about her sister. To me, this is a funny joke, but I hurt her feelings. I apologize and learn my lesson that not everyone grew up with dark, negative humour.

Journal Entry: January 2008

I think I am depressed again. I am in a bad mood and beat myself up over every little thing. Everything is my fault, that's how I feel. Am I becoming egocentric and self-centred, or am I retreating into my shell? I don't have a therapist anymore; I don't want to worry my grandparents. I guess I just have to deal with it myself.

My roommate, Jane, and I both learn a lot of lessons this year. We enjoy our time together. We are both trying to lose weight and bring most meals upstairs to be sorted into what we can and cannot eat. We can remove a chicken breast from the bun of a chicken burger, and we frequently get salads from the salad bar. One day, I returned from class to find the kitchen covered with chocolate protein shake and a note apologizing that she would clean up when she returns home from placement. It turns out, in her morning rush, she had removed the wrong end of the blender and the shake sprayed all over the kitchen. I am not mad. I laugh and help her clean it up when she returns home shortly after me.

During second year, I tutor a few classmates through the school tutoring services. Students pay a nominal fee to the campus service and get ten hours, which we initial to confirm we have completed them. I get paid by the hour and they get discounted tutoring sessions. I am excelling at the OT portion of the program, and I am often explaining concepts to the other students. Our professor does not appear to be doing well himself, and he increasingly struggles to explain concepts to the class. I get a huge confidence boost when others ask me to explain something.

I am hurt when a few of the other students call me a name in the elevator; it means teacher's pet. They say this after I ask if we are supposed to wear our OTA/PTA t-shirt to class this semester. I am hurt at first, but then decide what is the problem with being interested in learning? I try not to let their words get to me, and soon I move on.

Chapter 11

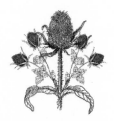

S PRING 2008

I receive a lot of positive feedback that I would be a great Occupational Therapist. I decide to apply to complete my undergrad degree in university to earn a BA in Child Health. Having enjoyed my brief time as an RA, I apply to Brock's residence Don program. This program is similar to the Resident Assistant program at Humber, which I participated in my first year. As I am not in St. Catharines, I receive a phone interview followed by an in-person group interview. On my way to the group interview, I am nervous, but excited. The manager sends me detailed instructions on how to get there, as the room is hard to find. Thankfully, I find it and am presented with a group of many other students, many of whom already know each other. I am the only one who doesn't go to Brock yet, and in introductions I make light of the fact that I am here interviewing for a job at a school I don't even yet attend.

I guess I make a good impression, as I receive an offer for a position as a Don before I am even accepted by my undergrad program. I get the acceptance email in class and let out a small squeal. It is louder than I expected.

"Sorry, just got an email... I got a job," I explain while sitting at my desk. I then backtrack and explain, "I got a job as a Don, not as an Occupational Therapist Assistant/Physical Therapist Assistant."

There are several schools I apply to and am accepted to all. I decide on Brock for several reasons: it's a medium-sized school, it's easy to get home to Pickering, and they have accepted me into their residence program.

I meet with my new team a few times before the school year starts in September. We have training in August, which brings us all together. My residence responsibilities are for two courts of townhouses in The Village. 'The Village' consists of twelve courts with fifteen townhouses in each, around a small square.

September 2008

My college diploma gives me several transfer credits at Brock, putting me ahead of the rest of the first-year class. However, they place registration for classes by order by the number of credits the student has, and therefore my transfer credits from Humber put me at the end of the queue of first-year students. As a result, my first-year classes and seminars are all at the worst times (8:00 a.m. or 9:00 p.m. sometimes). I have several classes with my residence students, and I form some study groups for my students who like to study in the presence of others. One of my teammates, Laura, and I start a habit of watching ER mixed with studying (one episode for one hour of studying). We make it through several seasons of the eleven-season box set before the school year is over.

First year, I live in a 'staff house', which means I live with the head resident of the team and the Don of Academics. We live in a four-bedroom, middle unit in the row of townhouses. The head resident gets an office and a bedroom, while the Don of Academics has the back room, and I have the front room. My bedroom has a large, south-facing window, and the sun streams in on sunny days. The bright light helps keep away the winter depression, and I do well this year. The memories of what happened in high school have faded. I choose to look forward with a positive lens instead of dwelling on the fear of those feelings returning.

The mascot for our courtyard of townhouses, called the "Green Gators," entails a green alligator cookie jar. When the mouth opens to take a cookie, it makes a noise. The previous Don handed it down to me and I continue the tradition of filling it with condoms, which we pass around at court meetings.

One day, I become violently dizzy and find myself crawling to the bathroom to vomit, then crawling back to my room. The room spins and I cannot stand up without falling over. A friend, an RA from another courtyard, assists me with walking to health services. They diagnose me with a viral inflammation of my inner ears. I spend the next week crawling to the bathroom and back to bed. I lose ten pounds because I cannot keep anything down. At our weekly meeting (in our living room) with the staff from our team, I am curled up in an armchair, wrapped in my comforter. The only man on our team helps me back up the five steps to my room when our meeting is done.

When the school year ends, one of my teammates and I rent a U-Haul to drive our stuff back to the Greater Toronto Area (GTA). I am in charge of driving the truck, and the drive takes about one-and-a-half hours. I am nervous, but I have others with me who can get out and direct if I need to back up. We arrive safely in the GTA. We unload all the stuff at our respective houses, and then I drop off the truck. I am happy to no longer be driving a big truck and shut my eyes for a few minutes as my grandfather drives us home in his car.

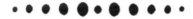

My home life growing up was not supportive. 'Sibling rivalry' understates the state of affairs between the children. Every comment I received from my siblings was about how bad I was and how much better they were than me. There was a term we learned in elementary school called a 'put down'. It means to say something with the goal of making the other person feel bad about themselves. This was all I heard. Playing my saxophone? I sucked.

Playing soccer? I let too many goals in. Do my makeup? I'm ugly. In fact, I heard so few encouraging words that when I began volunteering at a day camp, I was completely unable to provide positive encouragement to the campers. I just didn't know what to say. I was doing a craft with them one day, and the only 'encouraging' thing I knew how to say was, "You can do better than that," because I was conditioned to responding with a 'put down' mentality and had no script of positive words.

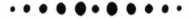

One summer, I take a road trip with my friend Sylvia. She is contemplating attending Brock but requires assistance to live independently due to her physical disability. We visit the residences and meet with the March of Dimes team to discuss her need for personal support (attendant) care while on campus. We discuss her needs and I mention I am considering applying to be an attendant, as I am a graduate of the OTA/PTA program. They decide to give me an interview on the spot. I pass with flying colours.

"While I would like to work as an attendant, I would not like to be scheduled for my friend," I state.

They look confused. "Why?"

"We are friends," I explain. "I help her on trips because I want to and I don't want to ruin a wonderful friendship by becoming her attendant. I will be her emergency backup, but I would prefer if you do not regularly schedule me to provide her services."

They respond, "We do understand. We can schedule this. Will you send a resume next week? We can hire you to do attendant work for other students on campus."

I have a few students I work with on campus who I become friendly with while maintaining a respectful boundary as their attendant. They are all accommodating with my hearing loss. For example, one student will text me when she finishes on the toilet, as I cannot hear her call. Another speaks extra clearly for me, as I have difficulty interpreting her speech.

Spring 2010

I begin to look for an apartment in St. Catharines and end up talking with a former Don named Cameera (who was a fellow Don my first year at Brock). She is searching for two roommates to live with her in downtown St. Catharines. My fellow staff member, Angelica, and I look at the apartment and decide to share the lease with Cameera. The apartment is small, but the bedrooms are of a good size and the rent is reasonable. It is upstairs and feels like a loft thanks to the railing along the hall by the stairs. The apartment is two blocks from the bus terminal, which means most months of the year I don't wear a heavy coat. I just have to make it to the bus terminal and into the doors at school. Everything from then on is inside.

My room is the middle-sized one and has a nice big window which faces south, so in the winter I get lots of light. It is a challenge learning to live with new roommates. I have lived with roommates for the past three years, but being in our own apartment instead of residence feels different. There are bills that need to be paid, a bathroom to clean, and messes to tidy up. We find a rhythm and learn to live with each other. Angelica is getting married, so I help her with her wedding invitations.

Brock offers ASL classes at various levels, and students receive encouragement to attend local Deaf gatherings. After moving into the apartment, I continue to attend the local Deaf events. My favourite is the Friday night social at Tim Hortons. The social is a three kilometre distance from my apartment and I cycle to and from it. I attend weekly and continue to cycle through the winter, donning my snowpants and snowboarding helmet. During the colder months, this allows me to continue to attend, as the buses do not run that late at night.

The local Deaf Community is very welcoming to ASL students. My teacher, Mario, is a community leader and often attends the social. At first it is overwhelming. While signing, their hands move so fast. They are used to students and will slow down to ensure I understand. I make two friends in particular, Lawrence and Amy. Both are a little older than me, but still on the younger side. They are very patient, slowing down and spelling words as needed. I pick up the language quickly. I improve my ASL and make friends, some of whom I will continue to keep in contact with.

I am talking to Mario one day after our ASL class about some difficulties I have in the classroom with the FM system and computerized note taker.

"You can ask for 'sign supported English'", which is different from pure ASL and not the same as "Signed Exact English," he informs me. "SEE is a visual version of English. It follows English grammar and adds things like 'a' and '-ing' to the words. You would not understand this kind of signing. However, Sign Supported English uses ASL but in a more English word order and adds more mouthing, and you can use a combination of lipreading and the ASL that you know."

"Thanks. You are saying ... to the increased exposure, I could learn many ASL signs through this method?"

He nods his fist in the air—signing, "Yes."

I think this could solve my problem. My ASL grammar and sign bank are not big enough to understand a university lecture. Using signs to support lipreading lessens my energy expenditure. I speak to our disability services about my request and specifically tell them in my email "Sign Supported English". Unfortunately, the disability office changes the name of what I am asking for to "Signed Exact English (SEE)", as though, as a disabled person, I don't know the name of what I actually need. As a result, they cannot find interpreters for the next semester, as university interpreters don't use SEE. When I investigate further, I learn that they have changed the wording. This is why no interpreters have accepted the job offer. My disability counsellor re-sends out the offer to their list of interpreters after they sort the misunderstanding out. I meet with two interpreters at the disability office and explain what it is I need. I can feel my energy requirements lessening as we converse in the office. We use this system for the final one-and-a-half years of my time at Brock.

Taking notes while speech reading or watching an ASL interpreter is next to impossible. I simply cannot look at something near and far at the same time. Even with a computer, there is a degree to which I need to look at the screen. It is mentally exhausting, simultaneously trying to look at the screen to take notes, shifting my eyes to watch the ASL and to process what the interpreter is relaying into English.

When using an ASL interpreter, there is the added stress of the inconsistency of attendance with some interpreters. As human beings, they get sick and have family emergencies just like anyone. Classes usually have two interpreters who switch back and forth, as interpreting is physically and mentally taxing. However, if one interpreter doesn't show, the other may have to work twice as hard. I can't blame them if they didn't work at all. They can't afford to get burnt out or injured, but sadly, it would affect my access.

Fall 2010

As my hearing loss continues to worsen, I make a name for myself in the Deaf community as a computer whiz. Soon I am fixing computers, and eventually I am given a name sign, which originates from the sign 'computer' and the letter 'L'. This initial name sign will evolve into the name sign I still use today. An 'L' tapped in the crook of my left elbow twice. Receiving a name sign in the Deaf Community is an enormous honour, and I am very excited to be given one.

It is also common for interpreters and Deaf students to become friendly. For one, they share a common language, and the Deaf student does not have to struggle with communication. Unfortunately, this can also make it hard to make friends in class. People don't want to interrupt or don't feel comfortable talking to someone who is signing. Sometimes hearing people don't realize many Deaf people can talk because they may choose to sign, instead of speaking during the class.

I often notice difficulty when in medium to large groups. If there are over three students, I find the conversation is fast, and that it is hard to keep up with processing all of it. This results in feeling left out. It is fatiguing to keep asking others about the information that I have missed, and I find it easier to just coast along. I would love to have the energy to advocate all day for myself, but unfortunately, the energy store just isn't there. My friends taking initiative to include me is what I rely on. They sign the words they know, face me, wait for me to catch up before speaking, and confirm I have heard/understood something. When it's dark, my close friends don't mind having a cellphone flashlight shone at their faces to help me lipread, especially if we are in a noisy environment. I appreciate when they do these things, even when I don't appear to be struggling. They know I am. I'm just not showing it.

Late Spring, 2011

Thanks to access through interpreters, I have the opportunity to apply to take a course in Italy for three weeks in the summer. I talk with the SDS department.

"If you are accepted, we will figure it out," the SDS counsellor says.

So, I apply. I write an essay outlining the reasons for why I want to go to Italy and I meet with the professor. I am accepted and then I inform SDS.

"I want to show you this," my assigned interpreter says, a week later, while we are waiting for class to start. She shows me her iPhone with an email out to see if any interpreters would be interested in going to Italy for a summer class.

I smile as excitement builds. SDS ends up contracting with two interpreters to go on the trip and an ASL interpreting student also joins us. This provides three interpreters for the three-week course, and then one interpreter and I plan to travel for an extra week to northern Italy.

I enjoy the course very much. I always thought of myself as a seasoned traveller, but not so much recently, due to the impact of developing a profound hearing loss. The access provided by the interpreters is fantastic. I have access to everything the professor, the tour guides, and the other students are saying. When I am not with the interpreters, I use a mix of speech reading and writing for the students with accents.

I am amazed by the history of Italy. I have always enjoyed architecture, and this course is studying Ancient Roman Art & Architecture. We visit many places around

Naples and Rome, including Pompeii and Herculaneum. Despite being a smaller site, Herculaneum is better preserved. I am amazed by the difference in architecture. The front of their houses have atriums, the part of the ancient houses I enjoy the most. I can picture them full of plants and water features.

I have always been friendly with everyone, and I rarely get annoyed by anyone, so I am happy to hang out with others from the trip who want to go out for Gelato or shopping. One evening, while staying in Rome near the Pantheon, we girls decide to take the white sheets off our beds and make togas. We take pictures on the posts and many tourists take photos of us. I'm not sure if they realize we are not part of the attraction! We think we are hilarious. The Italians probably do not agree.

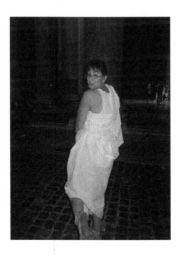

One day while walking down a narrow street, the rest of the group is slightly ahead, and I am looking around.

Suddenly, one interpreter comes over to me quickly and pulls me to the side of the road. I hadn't noticed a small van behind me beeping its horn, and the men were yelling, trying to get me to move out of the way! Oops!

Chapter 12

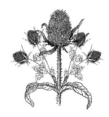

S UMMER 2011

In 2011, I apply for a Hearing Ear Dog during the summer from the Lions Foundation of Canada Dog Guides. I also find new roommates. My friends Julie and Megan agree to move in, and we get along well. Julie goes back to Toronto often, and Megan has just moved out from home.

October 2011

I receive word from the Lions Foundation of Canada Dog Guides school in Oakville that I am accepted for a hearing service dog. I do not have a car, but thankfully a local woman named Diane, who has a Hearing Ear dog named Spirit, gives me a ride. I am thankful for her kindness in dropping me off and picking me (and the new dog) up after graduation.

At the school, I learn how to handle a dog and keep up a service dog's skills. I learn about the laws for service dogs and their expected behaviour. We practice with dogs in training for the first two days. There are a few different dogs we practice with, but I fall in love with a male Golden Retriever named "Happy". However, he is in the Special Skills Dog program (dogs for people with physical disabilities) and won't be my dog. On the third day, we are to receive our personal dogs. There is a class of SSD handlers at the school, and they have already received their dogs. We make friends with the humans and learn to leave the service dogs alone to do their bonding with their handlers.

The trainers have us wait in our bedrooms (private, with a small bathroom), and I can see feet (both human and canine) walk along the bottom of the door. The anticipation builds until eventually it is my turn, and the trainers come in with a small Golden Retriever. I learn she is Happy's sister, Hilton. She is thrilled and excited to meet me. We cuddle and bond on the floor. I am so happy. Before long, we are called back to the classroom, where we teach our dogs to settle by our sides. In my class there are four of us, all women. One older woman, one middle-aged woman, and a younger girl the same age as me, named Sophia. Sophia and I are both in university and need bigger dogs that can keep up with us. The dogs are a black standard poodle, a black miniature poodle, a yellow lab (Cosmo), and Hilton, a Golden Retriever. During our classes, the trainer will teach and demonstrate, while another person types what is being said on a screen. This helps us, as we all have various levels of hearing loss. The other younger girl, Sophia (who gets Cosmo), was born deaf and knows ASL. We use ASL a bit but try to include everyone at meals (including the three people in the Special Skills Dog class) and speak and read lips. I become good friends with two of the other students, Cosmo's handler Sophia and a lady in the SSD class, Pat, who has a black lab named Sally.

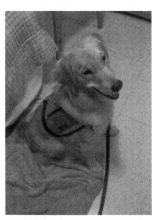

At the end of the two weeks, we have a graduation ceremony with both classes, our families, and the foster families for the dogs. My grandparents come to the ceremony. They are so happy to meet Hilton as well. It is far for them to drive, and they stay in a hotel overnight. Hilton's foster family is there, and she is as happy to see them as they are of her. Also in attendance is a lady from the Freedom 55 office (a business for retirement planning) who sponsored Hilton. The lady who drove me to the school, Diane, and her service dog, Spirit, attend as well. She drives Hilton and I home. I am very excited to have Hilton coming home with me.

When we get home, my roommates come out with a gift for Hilton. It's a dog towel and toy, and they are excited to meet her after hearing so much about her. They are very good about ignoring her in the house, as we spoke about this before I left. It is important for my roommates to ignore Hilton in the house for many reasons. One is that as a service dog, her bond needs to be with me, so she cannot become attached to others in the house. Secondly, she needs to always be by my side. Finally, if something distracts her, she may not respond to an alert, which could put me at risk. Hilton responds to many sounds and alerts me to them. She tells me about the fire alarm, my morning alarm, the kitchen timer, the microwave, the dryer. She will also alert me if someone knocks at the door and can alert me if someone calls my name repeatedly. At playtime, we go across the street and play in the parking lot with a leash tied to the light post. My roommates and I play with her here. They are in love with her, just as much as I am.

It is different learning to go everywhere with a dog. It's a little like having a toddler, as I have an entire list of things I need to bring: food, water, bowl, clean up kit, towel to settle on, etc. Then there are always people who come up and try to pet her despite her service dog vest. There are many ESL (English Second Language) students at Brock. Every so often, one of them will shriek and step back at the sight of her, even though she is not paying attention to them.

One day, soon after I come home with Hilton, I am waiting for a classroom to open. There are no seats, so I sit on the floor. Hilton comes and sits curled up on my lap. I'm not sure why she does this, and it will be the only time she ever does it, but I love it.

Not long after I get Hilton, I fall asleep on the couch, and when I wake up, Hilton is limping a bit. I'm not sure what she has done, but I decide to wait until morning, as the vet is closed now. However, the next morning she is not feeling well, and she has peed her bed. I call the vet and try to get an appointment later today. Diane offers to give us a ride so Hilton doesn't have to take the bus.

The vet is a wonderful woman who treats Hilton like she is her own. She gets down on the floor with her and checks her. I'm not sure what she says the problem is, but she gives me some Metacam, a pain reliever for dogs.

"Give her this for a few days. She will be better," the vet speaks, looking at me.

She also gives Hilton a shot of pain medication. The vet does not charge me a penny.

"Thank you, thank you!" I say over and over.

Diane drives Hilton and I home. I'm not sure whether to bring her home with me to my grandparent's house this weekend or not. My roommates offer to watch her, but in the end, I decide to bring her home with me.

Hilton and my grandparents very much like each other. When we get home to Pickering, she wants to go racing in to see them. It feels acceptable for Hilton to say hi because I no longer live at home. We have a routine—I bring her in on her leash and then my grandparents sit in their recliners to prevent her from knocking them over. I release her and she goes barrelling down to the family room, super excited to see them. My grandparent's love her very much, and sometimes I wonder if they are more excited to see her than me!

I have also been working for March of Dimes as an Outreach Attendant since my second year, when I lived at Quarry View Residence. Things become a bit more complicated with Hilton, and while she is okay to come to some of my regular clients in the University residences, it is difficult getting work beyond them in the community. People either already have a dog in their home, or they do not want a dog in their home. Either way, I end up not being able to work much in people's homes if I want to bring Hilton.

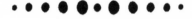

Early 1997

When I was a child, on Sunday evenings we had dinner at my grandparents. My Gran cooked an enjoyable meal, and after dinner, my siblings and I would go downstairs to watch *The Simpsons*. We were at my grandparent's house when we learned of Princess Diana's death. All the stations changed from regular programming to the news.

One Sunday night, after several years of battling cancer, my mom shared at the table with the kids and my grandparents that there was nothing more the doctors could do for her. She broke down crying. I did nothing. That evening, when we were alone in the family room, I asked her how long she had. She said six months, but in the end, it was more like six weeks.

In one of my last memories of my mom, they had moved her to a hospital bed in the dining room on the main floor. I woke up early one morning, knowing something was wrong, and went downstairs to see her distressed. She was mumbling in her sleep, agitated. My dad was in the shower, so I banged on the door and he came to her bedside. We sat there, my dad reassuring her that Liz was here, as was he. This is my last memory of her.

When my mom died, I was playing at my best friend's house. Her parents got a call, and they told me my grandfather was coming to pick me up. My gut knew then what had happened. My grandfather brought me home and everyone was on the front lawn, crying. We moved into my sisters' and my shared bedroom and sat on our beds. Everyone else was crying, but not me. I was shocked and numb, but felt I needed to be strong and not cry.

The first night after my mom passed, I was crying in bed. My dad heard me and opened the door. He sat beside me and rubbed my back until I fell asleep. The next night, I was crying again. My dad opened the door, but this time he looked at me, closed the door, and walked away. I'm not sure what his motivation was for doing this. Was he angry at me for crying? Sad that I had lost

my mom? Tired of dealing with us children? I tried not
to shed another tear after that.

After my mom died, we never discussed her death. I
guess my dad didn't know how to grieve himself, and to
that end he never taught us how.

It won't be until I'm in my thirties that I learn on
what day she died (October 18th, 1997) and how old
she was when she died (thirty-seven). She died on my
grandmother's birthday, and every year following, we
celebrate Gran's birthday with no recognition of the
death of my mother.

• • • • • • • • • •

October 1997

The funeral was in a big funeral home in Pickering,
and many people attended. I insisted on wearing black
every day, even though I only owned one black dress.
I wore it for all visitation nights and for the service.
During the visitation, there were quite a few kids, and we
were bored, accordingly we played hide and seek. Despite
being the only group in the funeral home, the director
told us we cannot play, and we had to go back to the
room with all the adults.

A few days after she died, we went back to school. I
surprised one of my friends by being there. She told me
her mom said I would be gone a few weeks. But I knew
nothing different. I didn't know most people spend time

grieving after a death. The message I received at home was "get back to life", so that's what I did.

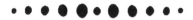

My mental health at Brock is generally not too bad. I have some highs and lows, and for the most part, I cope with it. In second year, while living in Quarry View Residence, I experience a bout of depression severe enough that I seek medication. I am prescribed escitalopram, but after about a week I feel hyper and wired. I putter around my room, up until the wee hours of the morning, bouncing between one task to the next. When this weird feeling starts, I stop taking the medication. I soon calm down, and I decide to push through the depression, as I don't want to risk that feeling again. I am terrified of reliving my teen years, and it seems that handling depression without medication will be more tolerable.

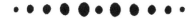

High school, 2002
My desire to become an occupational therapist gave me a bit of drive and a reason to put forth more effort in school. Up to this point, I had basically surfed my way

through school, doing the bare minimum. Despite this, I had decent grades. I took advanced math courses but did none of the work. My teachers hated that all I did was mostly pay attention in class and not do the homework, yet I passed the tests. One class used a T51 graphing calculator (do kids use those anymore?) and often found myself showing the teacher how to do various things on it.

Navigating technology and using computers has always come easily to me. My family has had a computer for as long as I can remember. Our first computer had a dark screen with white text; I remember my mom helping me to type an assignment using it. Then we had a computer with the Berenstein Bears computer game. (I knew to turn it on and type c://papabear to bring up the game before learning the whole alphabet). We then got another computer and were one of the first people I knew who had internet—"dial up!" My dad had a fax machine that saved to the computer. Our voicemail was also on the computer, and so we each had our own voicemail box ('press one for Liz' kind of thing). Our library had an online command-prompt type catalogue program, which I was the only one who knew how to access from our home.

I used the computer often, and I often broke it. This resulted in me having to fix it before my dad got home, and as a result, I developed quite a knack for fixing computers. In grade nine, I taught myself HTML so I could build a website. It was fairly basic and only had pictures of my friends taken in class with a stealth camera that looked kind of like a voice recorder. I was the only one who ever visited the page, but I am still proud of it.

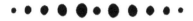

In 2011, I apply for a job in the computer lab at Brock. I am given an interview and do fairly well, but I am very clear at the end that I cannot hear on the phone and cannot do any phone work. I figure I have lost my chance and will not get a call (email) back.

Following the interview, the two managers have me do a series of common computer tasks which could come up while working with students in the computer lab. They are some basic tasks like creating a Word document with a title page and creating an Excel spreadsheet with charts. I have no problem and fly through the tasks easily. When I raise my hand, the supervisor comes over and asks me,

"Do you have a question?"

"No," I respond, "I'm done."

I have done it so quickly that he has a look of shock on his face. The supervisor checks my work.

"You can go," he dismisses me.

I never expect to get a call (email) back, assuming that my inability to hear on the phone has cost me the job.

Surprisingly, I get an email.

"Hello Liz, we would like to offer you a position as Lab Attendant."

The managers and supervisor are so impressed with me, they are willing to find a way to accommodate me.

I later learn that they had contacted the head of the accessibility department for the university, Nicole, (who I had spoken with previously on another matter) on how they could accommodate me despite not being able to hear on the phone.

The managers contact the Canadian Hearing Society, who come out to assess the situation. They are familiar with my case and know that I cannot hear on the phone as Bluetooth devices do not work with my hearing loss. So, they switch gears and install an analogue phone line at both service desks with a VCO/TTY[6], from which I can check voice mails. I'm not sure I will ever use it, as I never work alone, but the effort that they put into accommodating my needs in the workplace makes me feel very supported.

Hilton also comes to work with me in the computer lab (aka The Fishbowl, as it is a room full of computers surrounded by glass). She dutifully is by my side when I travel to assist students. One of my proudest moments is when I recover a file for a group of students that had spent the last three hours preparing. They had saved it as a temp file, but I am able to recover it for them in about 10 minutes. I have never seen a more thankful group of students. After helping them to save it properly, I leave them to finish their project with a smile on my face.

During my final year at Brock, my manager calls me into her office. I have applied to be a supervisor and they really want to hire me and another staff member. They have asked, but unfortunately HR says they can only hire one person, and the other staff member has slightly more management experience than me and therefore he will get the position. However, they can offer me a summer position working at the help desk. This is a privilege because students who are taking summer classes get priority for these positions. As I am graduating, I have completed my coursework, so I am thankful for the summer job.

I enjoy my work at the help desk. There are always two of us, so whomever I am working with will manage the phone, and I will take any walk-ups and help with the online chat. The system works well, and we make a good team.

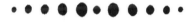

High school, 2002

In high school, I volunteered in the self-contained special ed classes. The classes had a certified teacher and a few educational assistants who taught 6-8 students. This meant that the class of about six to eight students had one primary teacher and a few Educational Assistants. These classes focused on teaching basic life skills (i.e. meal planning and preparation, simple writing and reading tasks). Since grade nine, I'd known I wanted to go into healthcare and was considering nursing. I got to know the students and staff well, and (I think) I was pretty helpful. I was very interested in assisting the students in developing these important life skills and enjoyed helping them learn basic cooking techniques. One day, an Occupational Therapist visited the class. She explained how her job entailed her to come up with creative solutions to help others to make life easier for them. One example was an adapted cutting board. I was hooked after listening to her and at that moment; I knew what I wanted to do with my life, to be an occupational therapist.

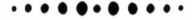

Spring 2012

In my last semester of my undergraduate degree, I am ready to apply for my Master's degree in Occupational Therapy. I apply to five schools, in hopes that by applying to more schools, my chances of being accepted will increase. My GPA is above the cut-off but not super high, so I am worried that I may have to do another year and raise my GPA. Thankfully, this is not the case. Two of the schools (University of Manitoba and McMaster University) hold interviews as part of the application process, while the other three are paper applications. The application mostly consists of; transcript, application, personal statement, and confidential references.

Hilton and I fly to Winnipeg to attend the interview. I meet with the SDS person who is in charge of Deaf services. Initially, I start to talk to her using my voice. She then signs to me, "Sign please." I did not realize the entire time we had been corresponding through email that she herself was also Deaf. We talk a lot (in ASL) about how they could support me, as they have recently graduated a Deaf doctor. They have a good idea of what would be involved, and the interview goes well. I am not a huge fan of Winnipeg—it is sooo cold in the winter—I decide to keep my options open.

Back in Ontario, McMaster University invites me to the MMI[7] interview process. I complete the series of interviews with the assistance of an ASL interpreter who signs the question to me, and I speak back my answers. After that, I wait several agonizing weeks waiting for responses from universities. I am accepted to four of the five schools I apply to.

The next phase is making the decision to select a school within a short time frame. I organize meetings with the three schools in Ontario that I have been accepted to.

I am surprised at how different the schools are in their approaches. The first school is very open to me attending, and I meet with the program representative and the disability services representative. They seem willing to work with me, but the town has a shortage of ASL interpreters currently and there is also a Deaf law student starting at the same time I would. Therefore, they are hoping to recruit ASL interpreters to move to the area. Being close to a provincial School for the Deaf, this is not an unreasonable solution, but it still seems a little less secure. The second school is not a pleasant experience. In summary, they ask me to provide my own interpreter, the representative from the disability services does not attend and they seem over confident to handle the first Deaf OT student in Canada. Three strikes and I quickly realize this is not the school for me.

The third school, McMaster University, is very accommodating. They have a large accessibility staff who come to the meeting. We discuss my needs and they openly admit there is a lot to put in place before September and that it will be trial and error. Finally, a school that is willing to say they don't know but will work with me. That seals the deal for me. I go home and formally accept McMaster University.

Chapter 13

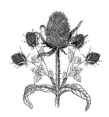

T HE SUMMER BEFORE STARTING my master's is busy.
I am working at the help desk most days and
figuring out school stuff the rest of the time. There are
lots of details to figure out, as no one has done the
program with ASL interpreters before. Both the school
and I get to work. We make it happen when I advocate
for what I need. I have to explain why I need all videos
captioned and that interpreters cannot interpret a video
properly; I also have to teach how to lecture with a Deaf
student in the class. I have to explain about interpreters
not being props and about pausing to let the interpreter
catch up before answering a question. We have to figure
out how I will obtain notes from lectures and seminars.
How will I function in a seminar with many people often
talking at once? I will need to write what they say, so
how will I do that while needing to look at the inter-

preters? How will placements work when I have both an interpreter and a service dog? How will the school approach the placements? So many questions need to be resolved before school starts. I enjoy educating others about how to communicate with me, including doing two presentations; one for students and one for faculty. I feel empowered that McMaster is fully supporting this and I feel like we are starting off on a good foot.

I also have to find a place to live near the school, as I detest commuting. I meet up with Jane, my old roommate from Humber, and we talk about finding a place together. We view a few dumps but eventually find a three-bedroom house. There is a separate apartment in the basement which is rented by a grad student. Jane has a friend who will join us, so together we sign for the house. It is small but affordable and has a modest back yard for Hilton.

While completing my master's program, I work twice as hard as the other students. Before each class, I review the lecture and complete the readings so I am familiar with the material. I review the typed notes every evening. I spend countless hours making my own notes from the computerized note-taker notes, transcripts from seminars, and readings. We (the program and I) learn how to make things work. The presentation I do for the faculty before school starts helps them to understand how to teach with a Deaf student and communicate with me without an interpreter present. I also get hired as the Audio-Visual equipment support. Prior to every class, I set up the computer system and after every class I lock it all up.

The stress weighs on me, and soon I find myself upset in the admin office, thinking I am doing a poor job as AV tech. I am reassured that this is not the case, and they even show me an email sent by one of my professors about how I fixed the projector when the IT staff wasn't able to figure it out. I feel reassured and vow silently to work on my perfectionism.

Seminars are a big learning curve for everyone. The students in my group have to learn to talk one at a time and let the interpreters catch up. They want to try a talking stick, which I think is childish, but if it works, I'm fine with it. It isn't long before we drop that idea, and the students get used to not talking over each other. We adapt in other ways. When reaching a consensus, everyone uses thumbs up or down as a visual agreement. This saves the interpreter from trying to identify each person and their response.

That first semester, I struggle with note-taking. Feedback with concrete examples is expected during midterm and final evaluations. I go back over the seminars days later when I get the transcripts, trying to identify who the speaker is (if the transcriptionist isn't sure) and noting the exact example. At mid-term, we go through our feedback, and I realize that somewhere, somehow, I have misunderstood the instructions. The feedback sheet has several sections, with several bullets under each. I misunderstand, thinking I am expected to provide one example per section, when really, I am expected to provide one example for each bullet. My feedback pales compared to my classmates, and I am told this.

I have difficulty keeping up with the extra amount of work I am doing. My grandparents have given me a small amount of money each month to put toward eating lunch in the cafeteria, therefore I have one less thing to think about. I try to go to the gym, and I get a locker to store stuff since I have both my belongings and a towel, bowl, water, etc. for Hilton. I soon stop having the time and energy to go often.

During the fall, I play soccer with a group of girls from my class. The first night, I ride my bike with Hilton. Despite her vest, we are yelled at by a staff member to get the dog out of the complex. After hearing that she is a service dog from several people, he relents and leaves us alone. Several of my classmates plan to complain to the Recreation department, although I'm not sure if they ever do.

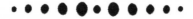

Elementary school, 1998

I was not very popular in my younger years at school. Shortly after my mom's death, a girl said something about my mom while we were changing after gym class. I reacted and punched her and the rest of the girls exited the change room, screaming. This was in grade four, just after my mom's death. I don't remember exactly what happened; I know I spoke to the principal (who was a friend of my mom), and then the next day there was a stuffed dog on my desk. It was suggested that I use it when I was feeling upset about my mom. This was the first time anyone had given me a coping strategy, other than telling me to "move on," when dealing with the effects my mom's death had on me.

I had a difficult time in school, and I seemed to get in trouble a lot, even though I meant well. But I was also stubborn, and when I lost my cool, boy, did I lose it. I recall one snow day (in grade six or seven), when they cancelled the buses. Since I was a walker, we were still required to attend school. Since there were fewer kids attending school that day, the teachers planned some fun activities (i.e. dodgeball in the gym). Well, I had not finished an assignment and my teacher forced me to stay in the classroom to do it. I lost it. Total meltdown. I tried to leave the building; one teacher bear-hugged me to keep me from running out. I was brought back into the classroom, where I sat in the corner on the floor behind the desks. I took a pair of scissors and tried to slit my wrists (not knowing, of course, that a pair of safety scissors cannot do that). The principal came down and talked with me, then my grandparents were called to come pick me up. The adults were all trying to figure out what had happened. What had upset me? Was I getting my period and hormones were getting to me? I don't think we ever figured out what happened.

This was the first time anyone witnessed my self-injurious behaviours. I started doing it around the time of my mom dying. I'd often tell myself, "I am bad. I deserve to be punished". Unfortunately, no one realized that this was not a onetime thing. As I was an active child, the reasons for my cuts and bruises could be rationalized.

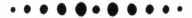

Until now, I have always dated men; I think of myself as 90% straight because I feel I want the typical family of two parents, two kids, and a dog. However, I know when I meet the right person, it won't matter what is between their legs. When I get to McMaster University, I develop a friendship with a classmate, and soon we are dating. We don't talk about it in public. While she is open about her sexuality, I am not. She is friendly, kind, sexy, and caring. She is learning ASL, and I meet her family. They are all very welcoming, but I don't know how to be affectionate. I have no recollection of my parents supporting each other, as I was too young when my mom passed. My grandparents are my only example, but it is difficult to learn from them when there is such an age gap and I have only spent a limited amount of time with them.

In semester three at McMaster, a random draw selects a small group of students to complete the semester in Northern Ontario (Thunder Bay). The program draws my partner's name, but not mine. She wants to discuss her three months away, whereas I don't see it as a big deal.

For me, three months is not a long time. We would text and I would visit her. I've never had anyone who cared, other than my grandparents in my late teens, if I was gone for an extended period. I have trouble wrapping my head around her anxiety about the separation. Eventually, she breaks up with me, as I cannot understand why it is causing her such distress. I will continue to regret this break up, and this begins my descent into another depression.

November 2012

In school, we are required to do four placements in different settings to learn hands-on skills. Collaborating with school staff, we determine what placements would be appropriate, and they approach the preceptor to see if they can accommodate my accessibility needs.

My first placement is with the Technology Access Clinic in Hamilton. Being a computer nerd, I am very excited about this placement. I bring a wire crate for Hilton, and she stays there when I see a client who is not comfortable with dogs. I do well at the placement, as it is very technical, but I receive feedback that I am a little 'odd'. My preceptors cannot give me examples, and so I brush it off and don't worry about it.

I show the OTs at the clinic a device I heard about which uses capacitive touch[8] to activate a mouse-like program on the computer. They are interested in it, as it is a low-cost device that could create a custom switch or mouse. When my placement finishes, my preceptors tell me if I want to do a final research project involving this device that they would supervise me. In my final semester, I take them up on this offer.

Late winter to Spring 2013

When my ex-girlfriend and most of my friends go up north, I am left alone for the semester. I have my spot where I sit in class where I can see the speaker, the interpreter, and the PowerPoint. Unfortunately, my friends who used to sit near me all go up north, leaving me sitting alone for the entire semester. I cannot move seats or else I cannot see everything I need to see. No one moves to sit with me, and this further increases my depression. I seek help from the campus health clinic, who prescribed me an antidepressant, Wellbutrin XL. I also speak to a few professors, who give me extended time on assignments. I have difficulty drumming up the energy for all the extra effort I must put into my schooling.

Late Spring 2013

My second placement is on the Complex Continuing Care ward at St Joe's Hospital in Hamilton. Hilton comes with me, as I have a crate for her in the office's corner. Hilton does not come with me to see patients. It would be too difficult to try to physically assess and transfer them with her. So, she stays in the office and I take her out on breaks and lunch. The OT office is tiny, and on the first day of placement, I am told where to sit. The interpreter who is present will sit in the office if there is space, or there is a small meeting room where they will stay otherwise. We figure out how to manage so that I can see the interpreter, but they cannot see the patient during personal care assessments.

I find the social requirements of working in a team difficult. My preceptor and I have different communication styles. I, as with many deaf people, am very direct. If I want to say something, I say it. However, my preceptor has a hard time doing this. She tends to 'beat around the bush' and not say what she is trying to say specifically. This is hard for my interpreters, who interpret meaning for meaning and are not always sure what she means. They often have to ask her to clarify her meaning.

As a result, there is friction between us, and I get depressed. I see a counsellor at the Canadian Hearing Society (CHS) in downtown Hamilton. I also see my doctor at the University and get a letter stating I am depressed. I won't give it to my placement coordinator unless I need to.

One day, my preceptor calls a meeting with my placement coordinator. She is finding that she is staying after work often. They ask me if everything is okay and encourage me to drop the course. I am upset, but I provide the letter from my doctor that I am dealing with depression right now. Later in the day, I have an appointment with the counsellor. I break down, as I am so worried about failing my placement. I also talk to one of my friends, who visits in the evening and we go for ice cream. Ice cream seems to help everything. She helps me decide to contact the school in the morning. Tonight, I cuddle up with Hilton and cry, as I am so afraid of failing out of school. Hilton has never been a cuddler, but tonight she allows it, even putting a paw on my hand.

The next morning, I contact one professor at school who I have a good relationship with and who also is currently the acting associate dean. I meet her in the morning, and she helps me process what is going on and to develop a plan. She encourages me to review the plan with my preceptor and clearly ask if I complete the plan, if I will pass the placement. She also does not want to see me with a failed placement on my record.

I go back to the placement that afternoon and meet with my preceptor. We review my plan and at the end I ask her,

"If I complete my plan, will I pass the placement?" Her response is,

"There was never a question that you wouldn't pass the placement."

I am both relieved and frustrated. Why did so much drama have to happen with calling a meeting with the placement coordinator if I wasn't at risk of failing? Why couldn't we have just sat down and discussed the problem? I realize this does not fit with her communication style, but I find it frustrating, nonetheless.

For the rest of the placement, I am careful to follow the plan to a 'T'. I pass, and on the last day I have an awkward goodbye with the OT and OTA. I give her a thank you gift; a mini rose bush to put in the window. A few days later, one of my interpreters lets me know about a meeting she had with the OT and OTA after I finished my placement.

"I wanted to give them feedback about working with an interpreter," my interpreter signed. "I said they had not treated you like any other student without a disability."

"How's that?" I ask.

"For example, the OTA complained that you always sat in front of the computer, and she always had to use the computer in the gym. I asked her why she didn't tell you and she had no answer." The interpreter shook her head. "I also asked the OTA if I was a hearing student and if she would have asked me to move? She said, 'yes'."

I still don't understand how the OTA expected me to know that she wanted to sit where I was told to sit if she said nothing to me. This whole placement I have felt like I am expected to mind read or figure out verbal puzzles to understand what is being said to me.

The shared house is not working for me. I need my own schedule to do tasks such as dishes and cleaning. I find an apartment in a walk-out basement[9] with a fully fenced yard for Hilton and lots of light. Another girl shares the apartment with me, but she rarely leaves her room and only seems to cook rice and fish. I build a garden in the back and plant a few tomatoes and peppers. I try to grow corn but that doesn't work well. Gardening gives me something to do to keep busy when at home and also gives me the opportunity for physical activity.

Summer 2013

In the summer, I apply for a job at the Bob Rumball Center for the Deaf in Toronto. The job is to assist the Sign Language Coordinator. Part of this position includes helping to organize the ASL Immersion Camp for adults. It feels good to be part of an inclusive, all-ASL environment. I spend the summer commuting to Toronto on the GO bus & train (intercity transit) and TTC (Toronto's transit system). Hilton comes with me daily, and I enjoy the ASL work environment.

The Sign Language Coordinator teaches ASL classes, and there is one class with a family who are learning ASL. The family taking the class has a young daughter with Down Syndrome. They need to bring their daughter one night, and the parents are taking turns watching her.

"Go join the class. I will watch her," I say to the parents.

Her mom hesitates for a moment and then accepts my offer.

The young girl loves Hilton. Hilton and I play with her on the floor while the family learns in class. Hilton licks her hands, and she screeches out, laughing. She has a wonderful time despite us not actually doing anything. At the end of the session, the family gives the teacher and me each a card. In mine, they thank me for my kindness in watching their daughter and letting her have a good time while they learn.

The summer winds down, and it's time for camp. I've been looking forward to this all summer, and it does not disappoint. I run around camp, setting things up, helping with the kitchen, flirting with the chef. We have a good time, but the chef doesn't seem to show any interest at the end of the week when people are exchanging numbers.

Late Summer 2013

My third placement is a paediatric placement in the community working with preschool children in day-cares and school-age children in kindergarten. I learn to work with children with various mental health concerns, including ADHD, autism or suspected autism, developmental delays, etc. As it is a community placement and with children, I decide it is a better idea to leave Hilton at home in the apartment, as trying to manage a dog when around small children would leave me unable to do my work. I need to rent a car for this placement, and I find one at a downtown car rental for a monthly rate. Since I have made good friends with my neighbours, an older couple, the man agrees to let Hilton out for a pee once a day. On the first day I return home and she's right at the door, all excited. I let her out, and she immediately runs to the fence and looks over, then back at me, then over again. She has this look on her face, a *Mom, you'll never believe who came over today* look.

Placement goes well, and the children are open to the interpreters. I also have a Roger Pen (a remote microphone) for situations where it is not appropriate to have another person in the room. Placement goes uneventfully, although I get the 'she's a little off' vibe at some points.

Fall 2013

Summer finishes and year two starts. In year one, I received a 'C' grade. In the program, you are only permitted one 'C' grade. However, this semester there are endless problems with my accommodations. I don't get notes in a timely manner and a bunch of small things lead to a lot of stress for me. So, this semester I again do not do too well in a class. However, the faculty decide to allow me to do extra credit to increase the grade since they cannot rule out my accommodation difficulties as causing my poor grade. I am forever thankful for this opportunity, as I know I put in more effort than any other student in the program, and I was born to do OT.

My roommate in the new apartment moves home to Toronto, and I make a deal with my landlord to rent the entire basement to myself. This suits me well, as I now have an office/guest bedroom and a bedroom for myself. There is plenty of light, and I can do my thing. In the spring, I even start my own seeds in a sunny window and again have a garden. It does well, and I make good friends with my neighbours, who also have a dog and a garden. In the summer, I enjoy sitting on my back patio doing work under an umbrella or having a BBQ. These little tidbits of self-care keep me going.

Chapter 14

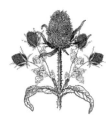

I LOOKED INTO COCHLEAR implants while at Brock, but my hearing had not deteriorated enough to qualify, and Ontario only provides one implant for adults. Rarely, someone could get a second, but it was never in one surgery. I have no desire to have just one implant. I feel it is too risky. I could do well with it, make a life using it to hear, get a job, a life. What would the implications be if it breaks? What if the internal components break and it takes weeks (or months) before I can hear again? I could not work, and that is not acceptable to me. At least with two implants there would be less of a risk of them both breaking at the same time.

I look briefly into cochlear implants in the United States just to see what kind of money we are talking about. I figure it would be about $100,000, which I won't ever afford. So, I put it out of my mind and tell myself I don't want it anyway, I'm doing fine as I am.

I have a policy in medical appointments to have the practitioner write their questions and comments. I prefer not to have an interpreter, for privacy, and I know I don't get 100% of the information when speech reading. Sometimes speech reaching leads to the practitioner thinking I have understood something when I haven't. Therefore, I ask the medical practitioner to write so that we both know exactly what I have understood.

Christmas 2013

During Christmas, a discussion around the dinner table leads to me expressing my wish to have cochlear implants.

"The family has discussed it already and has agreed to fundraise the money, if you want to get them," my aunt cheerfully says, to my surprise. "All you have to do is say yes."

I am shocked. I don't know what to say.

"Thank you. I will look into it," I say.

My aunt, who lives in Boston, helps me arrange for testing at the Massachusetts Eye and Ear Institute when I visit her in Boston. After a bunch of tests, the surgeon declares me a candidate. I pick the brand of cochlear implant I want, and they will figure out a price. I choose the brand Advanced Bionics.

I go back to my aunt's house and we discuss my results.

"I feel good about this hospital and surgeon, and I am interested in going ahead," I shared with her.

When I return to Canada, I email their representative:

I am a student, we will be fundraising the money to pay for the implants, and payment will be made with cash equivalent.

He replies a few days later with a price: $92,500 total. I discuss the price with my family. We agree this is a good and reasonable price based on my internet research.

"The surgeon also said he will do both implants in one surgery, since I have little usable hearing to fall back on anyway," I share with my family.

I discuss this with the school, who agree to find me a placement for my final internship rotation that starts later so that I can have the surgery before my final placement.

May 29, 2014

I have simultaneous bilateral cochlear implant surgery in Boston, Massachusetts. My aunt drives me to the hospital early in the morning, as I am the first on the schedule. I am very nervous but do not want her to stay, so she goes to work at MIT a few blocks away. I am met by an ASL interpreter, who stays with me until I am put to sleep. He is very compassionate. He distracts me by telling me a story while a nurse is putting in my IV. I remember transferring to the surgery table and then nothing. No mask to the face like you see on TV. They must have put me out through the IV.

I wake up in recovery with the feeling of compression sleeves on my legs. Inflate, deflate. Inflate, deflate. There is a different ASL interpreter, a woman, this time. I am in a lot of pain but try to stay strong. I have tears running down my face as I sit up. I am fighting the pain. The nurses call the anaesthetist, who orders more pain medication. My tears stop and I become more alert. Someone calls my aunt to come sit with me. The doctor had anticipated a longer surgery, so my aunt is in a meeting when her phone rings.

As I become more aware, I can feel the implants in my ears, even though everyone insists that's impossible. I can feel the electronics on my skull, and I am sure I can feel the electrode as well.

"Was it successful?" I ask the surgeon as he walks up—I speak with my hands.

The interpreter relays my question to him.

"Yes, it was successful," he replies.

"Why are you not talking?" my aunt asks me, through the interpreter.

"My jaw is very sore, particularly on the left side," I explain, in ASL, even though I am still slightly dazed.

I will learn later that this soreness is because of the location of the implant being positioned under the muscles of my jaw.

My aunt drives us back to her house. My cousin, who has taken a level 1 ASL course, becomes my relay. I sleep the first two nights on the couch with a neck pillow, as I cannot sleep on either side. Two days later, I fly back to Canada and jump back into school. I am no longer wearing hearing aids, as the implant has destroyed what little hearing I had left. I still lipread well, so I make do. Six weeks pass before I am activated. Typically, they activate patients after four weeks, but it fits better with my school schedule to do it at six weeks. This way I can spend a longer period in the States and have several adjustments (called 'mappings') before flying home.

July 2, 2014

The day of activation, I am excited but anxious. My aunt and my cousin accompany me on the train to the centre of Boston. At the hospital, there is an ASL interpreter waiting to interpret for me. The audiologist runs through the equipment and shows me how to locate the magnet on my skull that holds the transmitter coil. She does some testing and I hear a few beeps. Finally, she turns both sides on together and asks me if I can hear her. I hear a series of beeps but no speech. I ask her to turn the volume up and she sets a series of programs for me to use that slowly increase the volume of the sounds I am hearing. We return home and the world around me sounds confusing. There are no distinct sounds until we are sitting on the train, and I hear a distinct beep. I jump and ask my family what that was. My cousin explains it is a bell on the train, announcing the next stop. This is the first genuine sound I remember hearing.

We arrive home, and I try not to get overwhelmed. It is time to prepare dinner, but I sit in the furthest corner of the living room, bombarded by the beeps that are supposed to represent sounds. In my head I think, *holy shit, what have I done?* In the kitchen we eat dinner, and my cousins play me the latest hit song on the computer; "Happy" by Pharrell Williams. It doesn't sound like anything other than beeps to me.

Over the next few weeks, I will fly between Buffalo and Boston several times. I have the boarding process down to a science. I know where to check in and who I need to remind that I have a service dog. I remind them that I need a bulkhead seat and they should contact the passenger next to me to ensure they are not afraid of dogs. I never have a problem. No one minds having Hilton in their foot space. I allow my seat-mates to pet her if they desire. I feel it is only fair since she often takes a bit of their foot space.

The entire month of July, I dedicate myself to auditory rehab. There are several iPad and computer apps I can practice with. I watch YouTube videos and I watch TED Talks (which have captions). Every single day, I spend eight hours doing rehabilitation. I notice improvements daily. At first, I cannot tell what the videos say, but slowly my comprehension improves. I go to bed and wake up the next morning, able to understand more. Sounds click; once I figure out what a sound is, my brain makes the association and suddenly it sounds right. There is a beep I hear in the kitchen, but I don't know it's source. Eventually, I figure out it is the sound of the cupboard closing, as there is a metal latch. Once my brain figures that out, it no longer sounds like a beep; it sounds like it is supposed to (a metal clicking). Another example is one night when I was walking Hilton along the rail trail. It is a warm summer night, and I am hearing beeps all over. It takes a while, but eventually I realize I am hearing crickets. Suddenly, they sound like crickets.

I don't want to fool anyone into thinking cochlear implants are a miracle cure to deafness. They are not. I do well because I have a young brain and I have auditory memories. Doing eight hours of rehab daily for a month probably helped a lot, too. But hearing with a cochlear implant (CI) is not the same as hearing as normal, even if I describe some sounds as sounding as they should.

I try to describe hearing loss as a picture, since most hearing people can understand it better that way. Try to visualize a picture; you can see the colours, the details, it is an adequate size for viewing. This is my explanation of normal hearing.

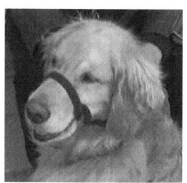

A visual example of normal hearing

Now imagine that picture has shrunk. It is harder to see; this is hearing loss.

A visual example of hearing loss

You can blow that picture up (as with hearing aids do sound) but it will become distorted. Colours may not be accurate or even missing, its size and shape might be off. That's why people with hearing aids still struggle, despite the added volume.

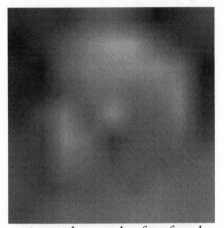

A visual example of profound hearing loss through hearing aids.

Now imagine this picture is so small that even blown up it does not provide a usable image; no one can tell what it is. This is deafness.

So how does a cochlear implant sound? First, you have to understand how the ear works. Our ears have a cochlea, which is a snail shaped organ containing tiny little hairs. The deeper into the coil you get, the lower the frequency of sound. A normal ear has about 15,500 of these hairs, each of which stimulates the auditory nerve. With some kinds of hearing loss, these hairs die off. When that picture from before becomes unusable, it is because too many hairs have died. With a cochlear implant, they insert a tiny electrode into the cochlea with a specific number of electrodes. In my case there are sixteen. The electronics can fire these in various ways to make 120 'spectral bands'.

To think of it another way, a normal ear-piano has 15,500 keys. It can play in thousands of combinations. My cochlear implant has sixteen that it can play in 120 combinations. Therefore, going back to my picture analogy, the picture of a cochlear implant is more like a pixelated picture. It might be the right size, but the detail is not there, the colours are probably skewed, and when I first look at it, I'm not sure what I'm looking at.

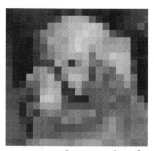

A visual example of sound through cochlear implants

If I have enough hints from the environment, then I can often figure out what it is a picture of. The next time I look at that photo, I will recall it at a faster rate. But I have to do this with every single sound, every single time. It's exhausting. Then throw in some background pictures (noise) and now I'm trying to figure out what it is when I can't tell where one picture ends and another starts.

Another way to think of it is like those talking pianos on YouTube. Basically, they are pianos that are programmed via computers to simulate speech by pushing keys in certain combinations in a certain pattern. At first you don't know what it says, but with practice you can understand what it's saying. Except that a talking piano has a full 88 keys to fire in thousands of combinations. I have sixteen keys that can only fire 120 ways (and most of those ways can only fire one combination at a time). So, the 'speech' from my piano will be harder to understand because there is less detail. With practice, it may be possible to understand, but it won't come easily.

Deciphering a sixteen-note piano, speaking all day, is incredibly fatiguing. I encourage hearing people to think of it as standing on one leg all day. Practice enough and you can do it. You might even do it really well. But after a whole day of standing on one leg, not even the best Paralympic athlete would still be standing and not be sore, tired, grouchy, and non-productive. So, if I'm standing on one leg all day, how do I get through it? By taking every opportunity I have to lean on a figurative stool or wall. For me this means using things like Bluetooth on the phone, a microphone in meetings, working in a room with no background noise, using a service dog to help with environmental awareness, and finally, sometimes I just have to take my processors off for some silence.

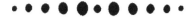

Early 2014

Towards the end of our second year, students choose our final research projects. I elect to work on the project I discussed with my Technology Access Clinic preceptors at the end of my first placement. It involves using an Arduino board programmed for capacitive activation, which can be programmed as a mouse or keystroke. Basically, it's a little circuit board we program to work like a mouse by moving a cursor on screen by touching conductive materials that are hooked up to the board. We decide to look at the idea of using it as a force-free mouse option for clients with Spinal Muscular Atrophy and Muscular Dystrophy who develop muscle weakness over time, which leads to reduced ability to move their hands and fingers. We recruit two clients to take part in the project, although only one finishes the project.

The project requires a lot of research on my part: I have to figure out how to write the programming language needed to make the device do what we want it to do. I also have to figure out some physics behind the device in order to optimize the technology. I have to complete literature reviews to see if anyone has done a similar project and look for research regarding hand function in clients with Spinal Muscular Atrophy and Muscular Dystrophy. With my preceptors, we develop a prototype board which has a raised dot in the centre and four strips of copper tape representing four directions on the mouse. We can use software to assess how quickly and accurately the client can use the mouse with various parameter settings. The benefit of the technology is that the client only needs to make enough contact to activate the capacitive feature, and we can customize it endlessly to suit the needs of the user. The device itself is also inexpensive compared to a traditional switch (the device was $50.00 US, when I purchased it).

Overall, the client likes the way it activates the mouse and that we customize it, however, being limited to X and Y movement planes (up/down/left/right) makes it less efficient than a traditional joystick, mouse, or track-pad. At the end of the semester, we have a poster fair, and all the students create poster presentations. It is all displayed on one day and it is one of the last times the class will be together.

August 2014

After a full month of auditory rehab, my final placement is at a Hand Clinic in Hamilton. I think this placement will work well because I can see my patients' faces, therefore speech reading will be easier. After a few days, I learn that my hearing has progressed well enough that I no longer require the interpreters in this setting. It is very different to be in a placement without the interpreters. I learn that the anatomy studying I did before the placement was not enough and I need to work to improve my hand anatomy knowledge. I find the placement challenging and feel that I cannot be as independent as I would like to be in my final placement. Despite this, I pass.

I must have been holding it all together, because shortly thereafter, my world falls apart.

Between getting my cochlear implants and starting my final placement, I get an interview for a job as an Occupational Therapist in Toronto. It is with a seating and assistive technology clinic, which is my dream job. The job became available due to a government grant. The clinic can hire someone under the age of thirty, and I am ecstatic when I learn I am offered the job. Unfortunately, this only adds to an intensity growing inside of me.

When I complete my final placement, I will be eligible to work and use a provisional title as Occupational Therapist. I still need to pass my National Exam before they can list me as a full Occupational Therapist.

After my activation and during my final placement, things spiral. My doctor tapers my antidepressant, but before long I am making poor decisions and getting little sleep. I must hold it together for the placement, but a few days after it finishes, I become full-blown manic. Much of what I do just doesn't register. I don't realize I'm not sleeping, and I don't see the safety concern of walking home from Walmart on the mountain to my home near McMaster late at the night. I walk through downtown Hamilton on a route that is about nine kilometres. At one point, I look at a big metal hydro tower and think I should climb it. Thankfully, something else distracts me and I do not follow through with that.

I develop delusions, which will become a common theme when I'm unwell. One delusion I work on is a number theory, stuff to do with binary coding, Stephen Hawking, and the multiverse.

Tuesday, September 30th, 2014

Somehow, I make it to a follow-up appointment with my doctor at McMaster. I am full-blown delusional and manic. I honestly don't know how I get myself there. I am writing furiously in my notebook in the waiting room and in my doctor's office. I remember her coming in and I look up for a split second to see her wide eyes, then I look back down at my notebook. She leaves and comes back with the psychiatrist and they ask me questions. I really don't care what they are asking. I must work on my theory. It is *imperative* that I figure this out. When did I last sleep? Saturday, I think. When did I last eat? Probably when I had Harvey's when I went to Walmart, so that must have been Sunday. I don't remember what else they ask. I think they ask me about my writings and I ask if they understand binary. They say no, then I respond they won't understand and cease my explanations.

At that point, they must explain to me that they are "Forming"[10] me. I must have enough insight not to make a run for it, as I know that would be the catalyst for the police to become involved. They put me in an office and assign someone to check on me. I continue writing, occasionally pacing the hall.

I guess they called an ambulance to take me to the hospital, because eventually an ambulance (stretcher and all) appears. I see it and proclaim, "No, no, no, no, no,"

I am not going. They get me to agree to walk to the ambulance and not go on the stretcher. I walk out of the office, up the elevator, through the large atrium, and out to the ambulance. My doctor has taken the time to walk out with me, along with a nurse. I'll always appreciate that she took the time out of her busy day to walk me to the ambulance.

I must text my best friends, because my friend Megan is waiting for me at St Joe's ER. They stick me in a room with a bed, a metal toilet, and a vast window facing the hall. I refuse to use the metal toilet in front of the window; I sneak across the hall to the bathroom. I also hide my phone when I see them take away the phones of other patients.

I'm not sure where Hilton is during all of this. My memory is not so great. I know at one point Megan takes her to a vet appointment, but my days are a little mixed up. My other best friend Bea, also comes to visit. She and Megan are a significant support. They visit a few times and even pack up my apartment for me because I am supposed to be moving to Toronto. Months later, I ask them what I was like when they came to visit me, and they say I was 'angry'. I assume because I didn't want to be there.

I spend a few weeks at St. Joe's. Immediately, I convince them to let me keep my phone to text as I cannot use the hallway phone. I have a Blackberry but no data, so it is my only lifeline to my friends.

Part of my illness involves not wanting to tell people and family where I am. I'm not sure if I am ashamed, or maybe I think it will put me back to where I was years ago. Eventually, my grandparents find out I am back in the hospital. It hurts them that I didn't tell them. I later try to explain that it was part of the illness. I truly believe everyone is better not knowing and I can handle this myself.

In the hospital, I am diagnosed with Bipolar 1—Manic Episode. The doctor's theory is that having my cochlear implants turned on has triggered the episode. I am, and am not, all at the same time, aware that this episode is similar to my experiences throughout high school. I don't have enough sense to be scared of what this will do to my life. Yet at the same time, I'm terrified of losing my new job if I don't get out in time.

While in the hospital, my mood becomes very irritable. I pace the halls, thinking and writing about my theories. We have group activities such as cooking run by an OT. One time we are making something food-wise, and I am trying to cut cold butter with some kind of dull knife. It slips, as the knife is not sharp enough to actually cut, and I swear my head off. Anyone who knows me knows that I rarely swear. So, for me to set off a long streak of foul words is very out of character.

"You need to go for a walk, and calm yourself down," the OT instructs me. I do, but I don't return to the group.

I have Hilton with me at this point. I have a private room with a blanket on the floor for her. She has food and water and I take her out to the bathroom and a few walks daily. I luckily maintain the insight and responsibility of being able to care for her while she is at the hospital with me.

I am given a cocktail of meds (Haldol, Seroquel, Epival, lithium, Zopiclone) to slow me down. It works within a few days, and I am left taking lithium and Epival to stabilize my mood. My mood goes up and down; I am well enough to take Hilton out for walks and bathroom breaks, but other days I am obsessed with Stephen Hawking or the 'third eye'. On October 9th, 2014, I draw the third eye and my thoughts on the sheets of the bed, not really thinking if anyone would notice the drawings.

My job in Toronto will begin soon, and I ask to delay the start.

"We can't let you do that. You see, the funding we receive requires you to start by a certain date," my employer informs me.

The hospital allows me to commute to the Toronto job for a few days. I am no longer on a mandatory hold, and they decide it would be okay for me to be discharged to Toronto. I am discharged on October 17th, 2014.

The psychiatrist advises me, "I want you to go to CAMH (Centre for Addiction and Mental Health—a large psychiatric facility in Toronto) should you need any services or support." I nod in agreement to go, if I need to.

Part Three

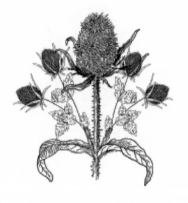

Chapter 15

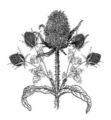

October 2014

I start work in Toronto, but I break out in a rash. It is red and itchy across my chest. When I call the hospital psychiatrist for advice, I can barely hear what she says on the phone. My hearing with my implants is not yet clear.

"Stop the lithium, as perhaps it is causing the problem," she orders. Before she hangs up, she repeats, "Go to CAMH if needed."

I am frustrated, as I am not getting much support or any answers. All I can do is hope for the best.

I am trying my best at work, but the hyperactivity and difficulty focusing are problematic. I have an appointment with the McMaster University psychiatrist (probably booked before they hospitalized me), which I attend, hoping the McMaster psychiatrist might give me a note for some time off.

"Are you seeing clients on your own?" the psychiatrist inquires.

"No. I am being supervised at work and not seeing any clients on my own," I assure her.

"I agree. Having some time off might help slow you down. I will give you a note for four weeks off of work."

"Is everything okay?" my supervisor asks, after I provide her with the doctor's note.

I hesitate for a second before confiding in her.

"I have recently been diagnosed with bipolar disorder and recently had a manic episode. They are changing up my meds again."

"I'm sorry to hear that. I will talk to the boss."

Coming off the lithium causes things to deteriorate again. A friend drives me, in the middle of the night, to the CAMH ER. I am admitted to the ER unit, and they try to stabilize me. I have Hilton with me, and they allow me to take her out to the grass several times a day. While in the ER, I receive an email from my boss at my new job. They are letting me go.

Over the phone my boss tells me, "You need to work on your health. I will mail you the things you left at the office."

I weep, harder than I have ever cried. I have lost my dream job, all because I have a stupid mental illness and a government grant that would not accommodate a disability.

In the ER, I have a bedroom and bathroom and am permitted to have Hilton with me. In the hallway, I notice there is something in the light. I climb on a couch, then a table, to try to see what it is. By the time I get up there, I can find nothing in the light.

After a few days in the psychiatric ER, they find a bed for me in an inpatient unit upstairs. However, they disallow Hilton from coming with me. I argue this decision, showing them their own policy on their website, but it doesn't matter. The unit will not take Hilton, despite her being a service dog. I have another friend take her to their home for the time being.

When I am admitted to the general floor without Hilton, I have a meltdown. I am angry; I am anxious, and things are going so fast in my head that I'm tripping over my own thoughts. I rage down the hall, kicking a bag of laundry. The nurse tries to get me to stop, offers me medication, but I don't want it. I want what's happening in my head to stop going so fast and can't understand that the medication is going to help.

"I need to go home. Being here is not helping me; it is making me more agitated," I eventually tell the nurse.

"It is the middle of the night," the nurse states the obvious. "So, we will have to get a doctor to come to the floor."

"Okay. Please do that, and I need an ASL interpreter, too." I am beyond the point where I can deal with sounds.

The interpreter and the doctor arrive. I take my CI off and just start signing. I must be signing fast, as the interpreter keeps trying to clarify what I am saying.

"I agree, you do not seem to pose a risk to yourself or anyone else and I cannot prevent you from leaving Against Medical Advice. However, I want you to know, I advise against this. You are clearly still ill."

Despite his recommendation, I choose to leave.

I take a taxi to my friend's house to get Hilton, then home to my apartment. Luckily, my friend is still up, and I can see my girl. She greets me happily. Perhaps she is a bit confused as to why she has been taken there. She is so laid back that she will go along with anything. Her familiarity and calmness bring me some relief.

The next day I tracked down the hospital ombudsman and made my complaint about Hilton not being accommodated, even though it says they will allow a service dog to stay with their handler, on their website. My words pour out of my mouth to the point that I am tripping over them. I can't get them out fast enough to keep up with my brain.

"Hilton is my hearing dog. Hilton is a professionally trained service dog from the Lions Foundation. Your hospital's own website commits to accommodating her and my needs. I can't hear! Hilton is a hearing service dog, not a psychiatric service dog!" I say, as Hilton and I sit in her office.

"I am sorry for the error," the woman says. "And since you are obviously still unwell," she asks compassionately, "May I call you a cab to bring you back to the ER? You and your service dog?"

"Yes." I agree to her assistance.

The second time I am in the ER with Hilton, they find me a bed in the Mood and Anxiety Inpatient Unit (MAIU). This unit is a sort of bent figure eight. It has twelve beds, all of which are occupied. With my thoughts still racing, they try every medication under the sun to slow me down. I see the walls bleed, and I walk around washing the walls with a washcloth. For some reason I am concerned about the walls being dirty, but the fact that it is blood dripping down them does not bother me in the least. I walk non-stop for hours at a time, from the moment I wake up to well into the night. Or, at least until the staff finally convince me to go to bed.

This unit, although small and the staff are friendly, is not in a good state of repair. For one, there is no hot water. The boiler is broken and cannot be fixed. The nurses try to get me to have a cold shower, but that sends me into further agitation.

The psychiatrist tries a bunch of medications. I cannot sleep, and she is trying to find medication to help me. One medication, Loxapine, knocks me out for twenty-four hours. I think I even wet the bed. Despite this, I am still wired. My thoughts are all over the place, and I feel as though I am tripping on them. The doctor isn't sure what else to do. They offer me ECT (Electroconvulsive Therapy, or Shock Therapy), but I cannot have that with the cochlear implants and have no interest in losing my memory, anyway. This is because ECT sends a current through your brain while they put you to sleep. It has some effectiveness if done correctly, however, it also causes memory loss, at least in the short term. With a cochlear implant, there is a risk of the current damaging the electronics in the implant, therefore rendering it use-less. Eventually, things calm down a bit, the medications start to work, and I am discharged. I start attending the day hospital program while on a multitude of drugs.

Around this time, I am supposed to write my National Exam to be an OT and attend my graduation ceremony. As I am so unwell, I breathe a heavy sigh and I have the exam deferred. I am very disappointed; I have worked so hard until now, only to have to delay the most impor-tant exam of my life. McMaster University also has its graduation ceremony, which I am determined to attend. I am not well, but I don't think anyone notices in all the excitement. Hilton walks across the stage with me in a little cap and gown that I have purchased for her.

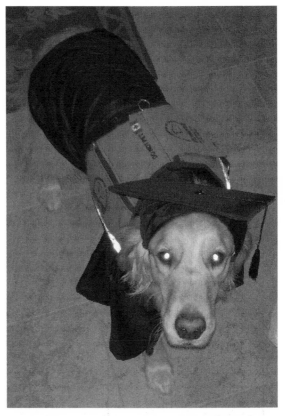

The Partial Hospitalization Program (PHP) is a group day program where you attend during the day but go home at night. The patients all seem to have serious mood or psychotic disorders. There is one man who talks under his breath non-stop and there are people like me in various states of the mood spectrum.

While I am a part of the PHP, I restart lithium. The doctors are running out of options to get my mood down, and at this point will try the lithium again, increasing the dose slowly to watch for the rash.

January, 2015

While at the day hospital, I attend various classes and meet with the doctor and other professionals. My mania turns into depression, and I become physically unable to move. The psychiatrist describes me as 'catatonically depressed'. I come to the program one day, walking very slowly, worried that I am going to jump onto the tracks of the subway. The doctor gives me a choice—call family to stay with me or go inpatient again. I called my aunt Anne, who comes from Hamilton to pick me up. She stays the night in my basement apartment with me, ensuring that I actually eat something nutritious. I think she sleeps on the love seat, but I'm too depressed to notice.

The next day, she drives me back to the day program. Again, I can barely move, and the doctor determines that I need to go inpatient again. My body and my mind are so slow that it takes forever to speak with the doctor and to get to the inpatient unit. It's like walking through molasses. I have a strange awareness; I know I am moving slowly, and thinking is difficult, but I cannot do anything about it. I can't physically move enough to take care of Hilton, and Anne takes her home.

I spend a few more weeks in the inpatient unit, this time depressed instead of manic, and without Hilton. My slowness resolves, but I develop odd delusions about Peruvian Pickpockets stealing my thoughts. I become very agitated, pacing around the unit. I get scared and steal a plastic knife from the dinner tray. I need something to protect myself in case they come after me and my thoughts. The drugs get me to sleep, but soon a nurse notices I am holding the knife and calls security. Two security guards came to remove a single plastic knife from my hands. When they come, they try to force me out of bed by grabbing my arms. Naturally, I push back. But this is a mistake, because now they claim I am combative and throw me (literally) into the seclusion room next door. I am not happy to be there. I quickly start banging and kicking the door, begging them, ordering them to let me out. I am terrified the Peruvian Pickpockets will steal my thoughts in this room.

I am terrified for a while until suddenly my brain gives up. I am not calm; I am broken. My spirit has been broken, because I have been secluded into a room that has sent my brain chemicals wild, only for them to let me buck like a horse until I give in and do what they want. I sit on the ground, my knees to my stomach and my head on my knees. I wait, numb, broken, until they agree to let me out.

The doctor feels that it would be best for me to move home with my grandparents. I inform my landlord that I need to leave my lease early and pack my stuff. Eventually I am discharged home on February 6th, 2015 to the local day program on a cocktail of medications consisting of Abilify, Clonazepam, Epival, Haloperidol, Lithium, Lorazepam, and Zopiclone.

February, 2015

My grandparents, once again, nurse me back to health after I move home with them. I need someone to get me up in the morning, ensure that I eat breakfast, lunch, and dinner daily. Reminders to shower and walk Hilton a few times a week are needed. For several weeks, I attend a day program at the local hospital. The material taught isn't very helpful, and I don't remember any of it. But getting myself out of the house helps me get back on a schedule.

At first my grandmother has to drive me, as I cannot drive. My thought processes are too slow, my reaction time too delayed. I struggle to walk from the drop off to the group room. In the program, we meet as a group and discuss various mental health topics. I attempt but fail to relate to the others, who mostly have depression as a reaction to an identifiable event. One lady has been hospitalized as much as I have. She has had ECT (the same as I was offered at CAMH but could not have), which she found beneficial. The other participants have a reason for their depression. For me, it feels biological. Eventually, I can drive myself, and I park on the street and walk across a field to avoid having to pay for parking.

At St Joe's, the social work student helped me find a family doctor in Toronto who had an associated psychiatrist. I see this psychiatrist for a while, but at one point I run out of medication. I can't get an appointment. For those few days, I seem to wake up; my thoughts clear, I show more expression on my face. My grandparents remark they are getting their Liz back again. Unfortunately, as soon as I take the medications again, I am back to no affect, slow moving, slow thinking. This is better than the alternative of mania or depression and being hospitalized again.

Recovery is slow. Some days I just lie on the floor by the fireplace. My grandmother asks if I need to go back to the hospital. The answer is always no. I take Hilton for a walk as often as I can manage. She has a yard to use for toileting, but she still needs to stretch her legs. Walks are hard for me, so I'm thankful that I have her here to force me out of the house.

I register for another sitting of the National OT Exam. It is in downtown Toronto, and I fear being late. I take transit and arrive two hours early. I sit in a coffee shop near the building, waiting for time to pass. Most of the applicants are international students or OT's who moved to Canada. In both exam sessions, I finish the multiple-choice exam first. As I have always finished tests quickly, I try not to stress about it.

In a few weeks, I learn I passed with a good score. I am now listed as having a full licence. This restores some of my confidence.

Chapter 16

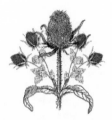

T HINGS START TO LOOK up. A classmate posts on
Facebook about an available position in home care
about an hour from Hamilton. I apply for the job, which
is about one-and-a-half hours away from Pickering,
where I currently live. I have an interview with the
therapy leader Mia and explain how I can do the job
despite my hearing loss thanks to my cochlear implants.
The therapy leader is a speech and language pathologist
and finds my speech amazing. I explain that I could hear
previously. I must make a good impression because I am
offered the job a few days later. I am quite surprised by
this. My grandparents worry I am trying to work too
soon, but I want to get my life back.

I look at a few two-bedroom apartments in my new
hometown and apply for the one with a shared fenced
yard. It's not huge, but it's big enough for a patio table

and chairs on a small patio and it has grass for Hilton to lie on and do her business. The real estate agent is representing the landlord, and I meet up to sign the lease. I provide her with Hilton's Lions Foundation of Canada Dog Guides ID card and explain how she helps me. I can provide references to support the dog won't damage anything (even though, as she is a service dog, I am not required to do so). It is not a problem, and I make a few requests before I move into the apartment: one - they get it professionally cleaned, as the previous tenants left a disgusting mess and two—to clean up roofing material which was in the backyard which could be dangerous for Hilton. The Realtor agrees on behalf of the landlord, and I sign the papers and provide first and last months' rent. The apartment is available on July 1st, 2015, so I need to find somewhere to stay during the month of June.

Mia suggests a student residence downtown in a near-by city about thirty-five minutes away from my new hometown. I can rent a room for the month of June until my apartment is ready. They provide me with my own apartment and only request that Hilton wear her vest while in the halls, as they do not permit pets. The apartment is for three students and consists of three bedrooms (two of which are locked), a kitchen, a living area, and a bathroom.

One morning, I take Hilton for her morning pee, when out of nowhere a huge, brown dog comes barrel-ing down the sidewalk at us. He attacks Hilton, unpro-voked, and I can hear her squealing. It is terrifying for both of us. There is nothing I can do until the brown dog's owner catches up and literally tackles his dog. I quickly rush Hilton into the safety inside. We go up to the apartment and I call campus security. While waiting for them, I examine her wounds. She has several wounds which are bleeding, but luckily, she was wearing her vest. Her vest has teeth marks, but they did not get through, thus protecting her from further bites. Campus security investigates and determines the man and his dog are homeless and other than escorting him off the property, there is not much they can do. They encourage me to file a report with the SPCA.

I frantically call a local vet and explain that I don't live in this city and another dog has attacked my dog. They agree to see her in a few hours, so I bandage her wounds as best I can and try to calm my adrenaline. The vet is not far, and he examines her carefully. He reports they are puncture wounds but thankfully did not rip, so she does not require stitches. He prescribes some antibiotics since the other dog is likely not vaccinated and reports that physically she will be okay. For the rest of June, I am carefully on the watch for the brown dog and his owner. Thankfully, the homeless man walks the dog away any time he sees us, but my anxiety never calms down completely.

In July, I move into my apartment in the Downtown area of the small town where I will be working. It is small and mostly painted yellow. However, I am happy to be in a place of my own again. It has two bedrooms, and I use the big room as my bedroom and the second room as my office. There are three small windows in the entire apartment. It is not very bright, but when it's warm, I sit outside in the sunlight on the patio.

One of the first things I do when I move to my new hometown is contact the Canadian Mental Health Association. I know I need help to find a psychiatrist, and I am hoping to find a bipolar support group. With CMHA, I am set up with a case manager, Caitlyn, who helps me get a local psychiatrist, semi-local family doctor thirty-five minutes away, and finds me a bipolar support group in Woodstock, about an hour away. I attend the Woodstock group once, but there are only two of us who show up and it is quite a drive in that event I do not go back.

Caitlyn is there to support me as I transition to life in rural southern Ontario. When I first meet her, I do not yet have a couch, and we sit at my tiny kitchen table. There is a door to the basement, and a centipede crawls under it. I scream and tell her, since she is wearing shoes, to squish it. She does and I feel so embarrassed, but I know there is nothing I can do about a bug coming up from the basement.

Previous tenants have neglected the yard. There is a goldenrod everywhere and a mulberry tree. Hilton enjoys the berries so much that one day, while at the Canadian Mental Health Association, she pukes a considerable pile of purple mulberries, right on the carpet. I put her on a tie out in the yard from then on during mulberry season. Next summer, I want to get someone to dig up some of the goldenrod on the edges of the yard. There are lovely daffodils and tulips that come up in the spring, and I plant some vegetables along the wall of the house.

My hearing is still improving, and I practice hearing on the phone. It gets better each time I make a call. My calls are usually very brief: I introduce myself as the home care OT and book a time to see the client. As I do this more and more, my brain continues to learn how to interpret the electrical signals it is receiving as sound.

October 2015

One weekend while visiting my grandparents in Pickering, I develop a severe pain in my shoulder. Assuming I have pulled something, I ignore it. I drive home in pain and discover when I try to go to bed that I cannot lie flat, as it is extremely painful. I end up sleeping sitting up on the couch, and the next day I go to the pharmacy. I ask them to help me pick a muscle relaxant, still assuming it is a muscle strain. However, the medication does not lessen the pain, and then the pain spreads. It spreads from my left collarbone, down my left chest, then across to my right chest. I still cannot lay flat, so I call our provincial telehealth line. The nurse on the other end of the line asks me a bunch of questions.

"You could have a blood clot in your lung, and you really need to get that ruled out," the advising nurse says. "I really think you need to go to the ER," she stressed. "Can you get there? Do you need an ambulance?"

"I can drive myself, as the hospital is three blocks away," I assure her.

By the time I arrive, I am sobbing with pain. Every breath hurts more, causing another sob, causing more pain. It is a vicious cycle.

Finally, hours later, I am seen by a doctor.

"Hello Miss Grace. I apologize for the delay. There was a child in distress," the doctor immediately addresses my long wait as she walks in. Being a small rural hospital, there are limited staff in the ER at night.

First, the doctor examines me and orders a blood test. An hour later the blood test, called a d-dimer, comes back negative, but she orders a CT scan, anyway. The CT is problematic, as it requires me to lie on my back, something which is extremely painful to do at this time. The nurse and technician help to lay me down on my back and try to do the scan as quickly as possible. I am withering in agony, as they have not given me anything for the pain at this point. I do my best to be still.

I am brought back to my curtain with my bed and wait for results. Eventually, the doctor returns to my bed.

"You have a blood clot in your lung. That is what is causing the pain. You're going to need to remove your vaginal ring birth control, as it could have caused the blood clot. Let me take a look at your legs again," she says, lifting up the sheet.

"What are you looking for?" I say.

"Signs of a Deep Vein Thrombosis (DVT), but I am pleased to say, I don't see any." She replaces the sheet. "I'm going to order a shot of pain medication now that we know what's hurting you. The nurse will be right back with it."

"Do you have an allergy to Advil?" the nurse asks me as she prepares the dose.

"I don't have an allergy," I shake my head, "but I have been told not to have Advil because it interacts with my lithium."

She puts the needle away. "I'll be right back," and leaves to ask the doctor about a course of action.

A few minutes later, the nurse comes back, "The doctor says, 'It's fine.'"

The medication provides a bit of relief, and I am given a prescription for a blood thinner medication to be taken for six months.

"Take Tylenol for the pain as needed," the doctor says before discharging me.

The next night the pain is worse and in more places across my chest. On those grounds I don't believe the medication is working. I return to the ER and after several hours; I see the same doctor.

"Weren't you here last night?" the doctor asks.

"Yes, and the pain is worse!"

"You just have to wait and let the medication work."

I go home and try to be patient. I inform my supervisor that I will need a week or two off work to recover. She and some of the local therapists make me a small get-well basket, for which I am truly thankful. It makes me feel less alone.

Early 2016

At the end of the fall, I join the local curling club, but as the new year approaches, my mental health begins to deteriorate again. The first sign is *the voice*. I am sitting in bed, leaning against the wall, reading on my computer. Suddenly, this loud, clear voice shouts, "Liz." I jump. Whoever's voice, it was crisp, clear, present. But I am not wearing any implant processors, consequently I know there is nothing I could have heard from inside the room. The voice slowly picks up, then becomes two voices, then becomes more. There are many—sometimes talking to me, sometimes talking to each other.

I start to deteriorate. First, I stop brushing my teeth, then I stop showering. I slip into psychosis and somehow end up at the Crisis Stabilization Beds (CSB). It is a crisis program for people with mental illness who require support but do not need to be hospitalized. It is a home converted to a six-bed residence for people who need to stay a few days to get stabilized. I have my own room and I am permitted to bring Hilton, as they understand she is a service dog.

From there, Caitlyn takes me to an appointment with my local psychiatrist, as I cannot drive. I don't pay much attention while at the appointment. The psychiatrist is asking me questions, but I am distracted by things I am seeing on the walls. I'm not sure if they are bugs or dragons. My memory, years later, seems to switch between both of them. I remember my psychiatrist picking up the phone, calling the hospital, asking if they have a bed, and then saying I have to go to the hospital. Somehow,

I (or maybe it was Caitlyn?) convince him I do not need to go by ambulance and the staff at CSB can take me.

We return to CSB, stopping by the staff office.

"I have a bed waiting for me at the hospital." For some reason I laugh. It's not funny, but my body and mind have decided this is the best way to deal with the situation at hand.

I call my grandparents on the way to the city hospital, which is about thirty-five minutes away. I do not want them to think I have hidden this from them again. The crisis worker helps me find the psychiatric floor, as I have never been in this hospital before. Once again, I find myself back on the psych ward. This floor is shaped like a T, with the nurses' station at the intersection. Bedrooms and communal bathrooms are the arms of the T, while the body of the T is the activity room, which has tables, a tv, and places to sit. There is a gym in the back hallway of the hospital. The elevators are by the nurses' station, but they lock them and require the nurse to allow access. There are men's and women's washrooms, but at least in this unit, everyone gets their own bedroom and there is hot water.

I become distressed at the voices and say (yell?) something to a nurse. I am given a pill. It is the first day I am there and do not know the procedure. The nurse does not scan my wrist band (which I do not yet know they are supposed to do). He gives me a pill, which I distinctly note is orange and oblong. The nurses' station has no record of giving me this pill, even though I can look up on my laptop the exact pill he gave me

(Risperidone). Having never seen this medication before, it is not something my brain could have fabricated. I meet with my psychiatrist, who also works at this hospital, several times over the next two-to-three weeks. He changes my diagnosis to schizoaffective disorder. I have a flat affect, with no expression on my face. I am tired and can't think. I don't understand the delusions/hallucinations are just that—the voices are an ongoing onslaught of dialogue only I can hear in my head. This whole time, my mood is fine and stable.

While in the unit, I run into an old classmate who is working in the unit. We talk for a few minutes.

"It would be nice to touch base again, and maybe grab a drink at the Tim Hortons in the hospital," the classmate says. A little while later, presumably after discussing with other staff, she returns: "I can't get a drink with you. But I assure you I will not access your chart, I will not discuss you with other staff, or be your OT going forward," she says before leaving my room.

I am left feeling a little awkward with her statements. In the end, she just doesn't come down to the unit while I am there.

There is a really sick lady in the unit. I figure she must have schizophrenia, as she talks and it makes little sense. Word salad, as they call it. She also grabs peoples' arms but not to hurt them. The staff treat her horribly, even though she is harmless. Is she annoying? Absolutely. One time she even tries to get in the shower with me. The single-stream-of-water-they-try-to-call-a-shower that hardly induces the desire to get naked and clean off!

There is no door to the shower, just a shower curtain. She comes in and takes her clothes off. I push the help button and eventually someone comes to remove her. The staff doesn't bother to deal with her the majority of the time. They put her in restraints when they are tired of dealing with her. It's not like she is hurting herself or others. She's being annoying and perhaps holding someone's wrist. It's hardly justification to strap her to a bed for hours and hours, screaming and yelling to be let out until they come in with a needle to knock her out. I am incredibly angry about her treatment. It is such an improper use of restraints. I search the hospital website, but they do not have a restraint policy posted. So, I call the hospital patient advocate and try to advocate for her.

Fortunately for her, she is gone a day or two later, but I will never forget the way the staff treated her. She is gone because a nurse has killed her. I can see him with a pillow over her face. The staff tell me this is false, a delusion, but I know it is true. When my psychosis resolves, I'll know this cannot possibly be the case. They could not keep a dead patient under wraps, but also, her door was always closed and locked with a key from the outside, therefore there is no way I could have witnessed anything.

During this stay, I develop the need to walk again, and I walk all day. It's an inner commandment mixed with restlessness. I must walk. The nurses ban me from walking down the opposite hall. So, I have to do more laps in my short hall. My iPhone measures 56,000 steps in one day, despite the phone being given to the nurses to charge for part of the day. Soon, my need to walk transforms and I am commanded to hit myself in the head. The voices have threatened to kill my family if I don't make a sacrifice and hurt myself. I walk up and down the hall, hitting my forehead with the heel of my hand. My forehead becomes red and swollen from the repeated impact.

Caitlyn checks in while she is on the unit as the CMHA county Case Manager liaison to the hospital. When they discharge patients from the hospital, the hospital will refer them to Caitlyn to assist with things like obtaining community support. Today, the girl in the next room is sobbing.

"Is someone going to help her?" Caitlyn asks during her visit.

"No, in a psych ward, they just let you cry it out. There is very little emotional support in these places," I report.

The doctor tries several medications. They seem to be making me sleepwalk at night.

"You've been walking around, trying to leave the unit," one of the nurses tells me.

I scrunch my forehead, trying to remember.

"We lock the elevators. We just lead you back to your bed. The doctor increased your benzodiazepines and Risperidone."

This continues to happen day after day until I am on a very high dose of Risperidone (9mg. daily).

Things improve enough after three weeks that I am discharged with the plan for me to attend the hospital day program. The voices are still present, but they are less bothersome, more like a radio in the background.

Chapter 17

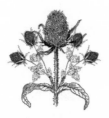

THE DAY PROGRAM IS in the same wing of the hospital, but on a different floor. There is a group room where we spend most of our time and complete most of the program. It is a large room with a group of tables with chairs around them. There are yoga mats for when we practice mindfulness and relaxation. Once a week we do an activity in the kitchen, such as making homemade pizzas. I am good at this, as I have made pizza from scratch many times, and I become the person who teaches others how to prepare and stretch the dough.

At first, I am driving myself to the day program, and the routine is good for me. But one day, it is difficult to stay in my lane on the way home. I hit the dirt shoulder and come close to the back of the car ahead of me several times. I guess someone calls the police. I arrive home before anyone pulls me over. However, the police see my car out the front of the building and track me down. They question me about alcohol, drugs etc. Obviously, I have not been drinking, nor do I take street drugs, and so they give me a warning to be more careful. This experience scares me, and the next day I take a taxi to the day program. My psychiatrist is not there. For that reason the doctor covering sees me.

Immediately she takes me off the benzos, reduces my Risperidone, and holds onto my driver's licence so I cannot drive. I am not sure how I am going to get home or back and forth to the day program. I call Ontario Disability Support Program (ODSP), but since I am not currently on income support, they will not pay for my transportation to the program.

I am very upset by this, and I share this with the group. Luckily, there is another lady who is also from the same area and offers to drive me daily. She drops her kids off at the high school just a few blocks from me, therefore it is easy for her to pick me up. She graciously drives me for the duration of the program, even after I get my licence reinstated.

This whole time, I am off work. I meet with my supervisor, and we discuss the steps to bring me back to work. Although I tell her about the bipolar, I do not mention the schizo side, as I am still leery about revealing any mental health issue given what happened the last time I disclosed that information. My work picks up slowly, and I resume working a part-time schedule.

For the next few years, I have various ups and downs of my illness, going between depression and hypomania.

Nothing too severe, though sometimes I have trouble getting up in the morning to work. My solution to this is to book clients later. Sometimes I feel fantastic and make not-so-great decisions involving spending and intimacy. I monitor my symptoms with Caitlyn, my CMHA worker. We know that when I'm hypomanic, I talk fast and I can't sit still. When depressed, I move and think slowly.

Soon, my psychiatrist convinces me to try the injectable antipsychotic called Invega Sustena. A nurse injects it once a month, and there is one less pill to remember to take. I have great anxiety about taking it. What if I have side effects and I am stuck with them for one month or more? I also have intense anxiety regarding the needle itself. It often takes two people to administer it, as I have an anxiety attack for the needle stick portion. However, the medication seems to work, so I push myself and continue to get it.

After a year, they approve a newer medication that only has to be injected once every three months. It is the same drug as my current injection, but it lasts longer. While approved in Canada, the provincial drug program has not approved it, so my psychiatrist gets me on a program through which the company will provide samples. When the Ontario Drug Benefit finally approves it, they pay the cost of approximately $1500 every three months, in addition to all of my other medications.

The injections work well at controlling many symptoms; however, there are side effects, most of which I realize were happening when I eventually go off the medication in the future. One of the most embarrassing is the drooling; not down my face but drips of saliva landing on my work. It's gross. I also realize (when I eventually stop taking the medication) that it affects my facial expression and personality.

Fall 2016

Throughout my life, doctors have had concerns about my joints, as I am always in some kind of pain. I am always getting bruises, and I don't know what makes them occur. My mom had ITP, which is a blood disorder and can cause bruising. While at McMaster they referred me to a rheumatologist, who decided I had something between Ehlers-Danlos Syndrome and Brittle Bone Disease, but nothing came of it.

However, after the changes to my mental health, I question if there is a connection between all of this and my hearing. My doctor refers me to a genetics clinic in downtown Toronto. I visit the clinic several times, and they run several blood tests. The first visit consists of them asking a ton of questions about seemingly every system in my body. The doctor takes measurements of my flexibility, my head circumference, looks at my jaw, asks about my blood clots in my lungs, and so on. I come back twice more for follow-up questions and more blood work.

"You have Stickler Syndrome, which explains many of your symptoms, including your nearsightedness, your hearing loss, your flexibility, and your bruising. However, there are no identified genes which cause mental health disorders," the doctor explains on my next visit. "So, I do not have all the answers I know you were looking for, but we have a bunch of things figured out." she tried to sound cheerful. "You don't have any of the breast cancer genes, despite your mother having breast cancer."

"But what is Stickler Syndrome?" I ask.

"Stickler Syndrome is a genetic disorder which affects the connective tissue, usually collagen. It results in many symptoms associated with poor connective tissue structure such as cleft palate, nearsightedness, hearing loss, hypermobility, heart and aorta problems, retinal detachment, early onset osteoarthritis, distinct facial features including flat face and small chin, and mitral valve prolapse," the doctor explains.[11]

I also attend the early breast screening program in Hamilton yearly for mammography and ultrasound (as I cannot have an MRI because of the magnet in the cochlear implants).

December 2016

My grandfather is admitted to the hospital in Pickering, again, with heart failure. He experienced a significant heart failure episode when we were in Boston several years ago. He does some more rehab this time, but we all know my grandmother cannot care for him alone at home. My aunt and I discuss with my grandfather how Gran cannot do it, especially given her new back pain. I don't tell them, but I have already decided that if they choose to stay in their house, that I am going to move home and help. Once we help my grandfather to understand that Gran cannot manage it alone, he says he will talk to her.

When we get home, my grandfather calls my Gran and they decide that as long as they are together, it doesn't matter where they are. My aunt and I look at retirement/assisted living facilities. There are some big ones in Pickering, but my grandmother doesn't particularly like them. There is a new set of condos being built in Hamilton in a seniors' complex, which provides assistance and also includes several meals a week. My grandparents decide on this option, as it will be near my aunt and uncle. However, the condos are still under construction, so they still need somewhere to go while waiting.

Everywhere we look, there is a wait list for the retirement homes. The only place we find that doesn't have a wait list is a newly built retirement home in my town. I tour the facility and they have a south-facing, corner, one-bedroom suite with a wheelchair accessible bathroom for my grandfather. I take pictures showing the sun coming in the windows and my grandmother agrees that this will be suitable for the short term until the condo is ready.

In January 2017, they move into the retirement home near me, five minutes from my apartment. We have the retirement home furnish the room so that we do not need to worry about moving furniture. I pick my grandfather up from the hospital in Ajax and drive him to his new home, about a two-hour drive. He does not want to stop by the house. I'm sure it must be painful to know he is never going back. The retirement home is a different lifestyle, but they get used to having meals provided and someone coming to help my grandfather shower and dress every morning and evening.

I visit daily, pick up groceries for them, and do the impossible task of finding them a local doctor. When I moved to my current town, there were no family doctors accepting patients, and I had to find a doctor in the closest city. For my grandparents, I draft a letter explaining their circumstances and fax it to every doctor's office in town. To my surprise, one of the best local doctors accepts them as patients! This doctor has an excellent reputation and specializes in geriatric patient needs. I am happy they now have a good local doctor and won't have to go to the city 40 minutes away.

My grandfather becomes sick again a few months later. This time, in addition to his heart, he doesn't seem to think clearly. He calls out to my grandmother at all hours of the night and day. When I visit him in the hospital, he introduces me to the stock shelf as his granddaughter. The nurses have moved his bed next to the supply shelf in the hallway near the nurses' station to monitor him. When he is medically stable, the retirement home assesses him and lets us know they cannot provide the care he needs. He is therefore put on a crisis list for a nursing home. He is fortunate to get his top choice, a home which is run by the municipality and just down the street from my grandmother. Part of the reason he gets a bed within a few weeks is that he can afford the private room. The way they set the bed system up allows people who are willing and able to pay for a private room to get a bed quicker, with the option once having become a resident of the home to have first access to double rooms when they become available.

For the next several months, my grandmother goes to the long-term care home daily, and I take her most evenings. My grandfather continues to deteriorate, and I accept he will die soon. One night, this hits me, and I weep alone at night in bed. This is very hard for me, as my grandparents are my lifeline. When I was told I was no longer welcome at home, he did not skip a beat about taking me home into his and my grandmother's care. I am determined to do the same for him, even if I cannot take him home to care for him.

Around this time, I look to purchase a house. A small, two-bedroom semi in a friendly neighbourhood appeals to me. I had hoped for a three-bedroom bungalow, but this two-bedroom semi is more affordable. With a finished basement, there is plenty of room. I put in the only offer, so I get it at the asking price. It is small but inexpensive as far as houses go, and most importantly, it will be mine.

My grandmother had previously told me that when she could no longer live at home, she wanted to live with family. She did not want to go to a retirement home. So, I renovate the bathroom with the intention of my grandmother being able to shower there if she comes to live or stay with me. I pull out the fibreglass shower stall and install a tiled, curbless shower with grab bars and hand-held shower head.

Shortly after purchasing the house, my grandfather passes, and I am so disappointed that he could never see it. The day before he passes, I go for a medical test that requires sedation because of my anxiety. I am advised not to drive, and for that reason, when my grandmother calls asking me to take her to see my grandfather, I say "Not tonight". The next morning, he passes. I regret being unable to take her, although I try not to feel guilty about it.

Chapter 18

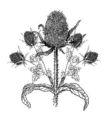

ON JANUARY 1ST, 2018, I decide to start seriously losing weight. My highest weight a few months ago was 192+lbs, and I am disgusted with myself. I join Noom at a sale price and work hard for two years. I get down to 142 pounds by the end of 2019 (my goal is 135 pounds).

Unfortunately, I become ill again. I am on my third case manager because of various staffing changes. There are no mood changes with this episode that I am aware of. I find myself totally preoccupied with my number theory and Stephen Hawking's multiverse. I once again end up at the Crisis Stabilization Beds (CSB), and I buy all of Hawking's books and study each and every one. I am taking more notes than I ever took on anything in school and am trying to draw my own conclusions. I spend all day and all night working on my theories.

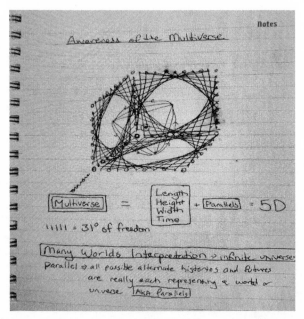

I fill my entire notebook with drawings and notes, and I care about nothing else. Thankfully, I don't need the hospital again, although I need to be reminded to eat and sleep. I improve with outpatient treatment, and before long I am once again working nearly full time.

I continue with a healthy-sick-healthy cycle for a long time. Meds too high? Hypomania. Meds too low? Depression. Lithium stabilizes that cycle to less severe swings, and now I no longer get to the extremes. One thing I notice with these episodes is a sort of 'hang-over' effect on my brain. Thinking is difficult, and there is a ringing that follows many sounds. Kind of like a reverberation or an auditory migraine. There isn't much I can do about it except push on and try to rest.

My grandmother stays at the retirement home, as she enjoys having her independence. She is not driving but can take a taxi at a senior rate to her hair appointments, and she has a friend in the home who drives. She makes several friends and takes part in some activities, like bocce ball. The retirement home has frequent activities, and she joins a Scrabble group with three other ladies. She asks me to get her a deluxe Scrabble board that turns and the ladies love it. They play a strange version of scrabble where they don't keep score but the winner is the first person to use up all of their tiles. My grandmother doesn't seem to mind and seems to enjoy the company of her friends. I think it is a wonderful decision for her to stay there where she has many friends to talk with.

December 2019

My grandmother and I are coasting through life just fine until we go to the United States for Christmas. On this journey, I develop a terrible case of vertigo and motion sickness. I am fine in the morning, but by the time we arrive in New Hampshire, I have thrown up in the car from motion sickness. The next morning, I woke up with a cough and a stuffed-up nose. COVID is not yet something we know about, so I'm confident, in retrospect, that it is just a cold. Also, no one else really catches it (my nephew gets sniffles, but nothing severe) which is not what would be expected with COVID.

When we return from the States, I discover I remain incredibly dizzy. I am driving for hours every day for work and suffering from motion sickness. I am initially told it is just from the cold virus and will go away in six to eight weeks. However, COVID hits, six to eight months pass and my symptoms persist. My doctor sends a referral to the Cochlear Implant program in London, Ontario, to be checked. The ENT surgeon sends me for vestibular testing and finds that it is not my vestibular system that is causing the problem. After speaking to the ENT in a phone appointment, he suggests it could be vestibular migraines, and he would recommend my doctor consider a neurology appointment for diagnosis.

This whole time I am desperate to manage with the dizziness and motion sickness. I find the only thing that helps is to eat constantly while driving. So, I pack super healthy lunches that I can eat while driving, grapes, berries, nuts, and I snack on these. The pounds come back on because of these extra calories. Never mind that I am walking Hilton several times a day, every day; I am still regaining the weight.

With COVID, many things change. The retirement homes shut out visitors, and my work gets incredibly busy. The medical system is desperate to get people out of the hospital and keep them out. Therefore, the demand for OT services skyrockets. They introduce rules about wearing masks, then eye protection. At first, this is an immense problem for me, as I rely on lipreading. I develop a script to introduce myself and explain that I have a hearing loss and may need them to repeat some things. I'm probably one of the few people in the world who benefits in some way from COVID, as it forces me to stop lipreading and makes my brain learn to interpret the signals it is receiving.

I have to stop seeing my grandmother daily, as I am not permitted to visit, and I take Hilton out even more since I now have more time. Rain, snow, sun—it doesn't matter; we walk. The only time we don't walk is if it is too icy to be safe or too windy that I worry about something blowing into us. Otherwise, we walk; not always long if the weather is crappy—maybe just to the corner and back.

I have been taking Abilify and Trinza for several years, but I still have so much anxiety about the needle. The injection is given every three months; it is big, and it stings. It leaves me with a lump of medicine in the muscle at my hip. I have so much needle anxiety that I have to psych myself up for five minutes at the office before I can allow the nurse to open the box. I can't let her tell me when she goes to do it (or I will flinch), and then the injection itself burns. My strategy to get through the injection is to count out loud to thirty. Sometimes she is still injecting at that point, and she'll instruct me to keep counting. Or sometimes the plunger sticks, and I'll get a sudden gush of stinging when the plunger moves again. I suspect the medicine is thick, based on the lump it leaves and the difficulty with injecting it. But I can never look at the needle and I am very clear that I am never to see it. The shot is expensive too, at $1500 every three months, thankfully covered by Ontario Drug Benefit (ODB). I guess it's cheaper than a hospital stay for the government to pay for my medications, but I have a heart attack every time I see the price!

During COVID, I decide I want to stop my antipsychotics and see how I do without them. My psychiatrist initially disagrees and reminds me how severe my illness is, but I persist, and he agrees to titrate it down. But when it comes time for the next shot, I decide I am done and I will not have it anymore. I will see how it goes without it. I'm sure he thinks I will end up back in the hospital.

Over the next year, I slowly 'wake up'. I hadn't thought I had many side effects with the Trinza, but as it gets out of my system, I change that awareness. My negative symptoms (like my flat affect and poverty of thought) improve, I think clearer, and my memory is better. Suddenly, people are friendlier to me (or maybe I am more approachable?). Everyone knows Hilton and I in the neighbourhood, but now we stop and actually chat.

Previously, I had no thoughts. I don't mean it like 'nothing to say', I mean it literally like 'there was nothing going on in my head'. I could not carry a conversation. I would eat dinner in silence when out with people, since I had nothing to say. "Poverty of Thought" I believe is what they call it. It slowly improves once I stop taking the antipsychotics, and now I no longer struggle to the same degree.

Easter 2021

Around Easter 2021, I notice Hilton is not feeling well. She doesn't want to eat her peanut butter No-Hide bone and for several days leaves her food untouched. I take her to the veterinarian, who runs a blood test, which shows high liver enzymes. The vet recommends an x-ray and diagnoses her with a liver tumour. He gives her six-to-eight months, and there is possibly an option for surgery. He doesn't know if her tumour is operable, and the surgery is $15,000. It would also have to be done in Toronto and involves a one-month recovery time, during which someone would need to be with her at all times. At eleven years old, I don't think that it is in Hilton's best interest to pursue the surgery. It is hard for me to decide, but I choose to spoil her for the rest of her time, and hope that I will get to spend the summer with her.

A few weeks later, she becomes even more ill, and thankfully my vet can get her in for an emergency ultrasound and consult in just a few days. The ultrasound shows a diffuse liver tumour (inoperable) and likely paraneoplastic syndrome, causing her symptoms. The consulting vet recommends prednisone long-term.

Hilton picks up with the prednisone. I also try her on various supplements but ultimately decide there is not enough science behind them to justify the $90/month price, and she doesn't want to take them, anyway. A few months later, I have to give her an appetite stimulant when she doesn't want to eat, and she has a whole medication-food regimen. I wake up at 5:30 a.m. every morning to give her pills, as they need to be spaced out around her food. She is not eating much because of the tumour pressing on her stomach, so I have to give her as many small meals as she will eat in a day.

My neighbour, Isabella, is a great help and lets Hilton out and gives her lunch on days when I am gone for more than a few hours at work. Isabella lives behind me and has a golden retriever named Bella, and her spouse

teaches me what to do with my yard work. Hilton is able
to keep on some pounds with Isabella visiting her daily to
feed her. This also reduces the number of accidents in the
house. Now and then, there is a pile of poop greeting me
or Isabella when we enter. We know Hilton isn't doing
it on purpose, so we don't get mad, just clean it up. One
time, she poops in the shower, which is super easy to
clean up!

Hilton's health slowly declines. I borrow a ramp from
my groomer to get her into my new car, an HRV, which
is higher than my old car, a Fit. At first, I don't think
it will work, but after a few minutes my groomer and I
figure out that she can go up the ramp into the trunk,
then I fold down half the back seat for her to go around
and sit. Then I can fold up the seat, put the ramp in the
trunk, and be on our way. It is not quick, but it works.
We also have to cut our walk distance in half, as she
can no longer do the long walk. She likes to go just as
far as a neighbour's house (a man named Wayne) about
600 metres away. This neighbour has watched for her
for many months and never fails to come out and give
her treats on our walks. Near the end, I hand him pills
wrapped in cheese and he gets her to take them, as she
has figured out that the cheese I give her contains pills.
In her last week, I can tell that she will not be here much
longer. I take her to the retirement home, and she says
bye to the ladies there. We also do one last walk, and I
make sure she sees Wayne as I knock on his door. I'm
glad I do, as it is the last walk she will ever go on.

On December 7th, 2021, I wake up to Hilton having vomited on the floor in my bedroom. She barely rouses, and I know it is time. I contact the vet who does the home euthanasia and my aunt Anne, who had said she would come when it is time. I send out multiple text messages and leave notes on several front doors of her closest neighbour friends. Hilton has many visitors that day: several neighbours from my street or the streets we used to walk by, my case worker Olivia comes to give me support and say bye to Hilton, and my aunt and grandmother come as well. My friend Megan wants to come, but cannot come until the evening. The veterinarian has asked for as few people as possible because of COVID, so I decide she doesn't need to come tonight, as Hilton will probably be gone before she arrives. Overall, Hilton has nine visitors on her final day.

My aunt picks up my grandmother so she can say her goodbyes. I think it is tough on my grandmother, as she has really become quite fond of Hilton. Letting Hilton go is one of the hardest things I've ever done, and one of the few times in my life when I weep.

"She is dehydrated, and she has lost a lot of weight," the veterinarian explains.

I do not want her to suffer. I would rather give up a few days and do it too early than wait too long and have her suffer.

The vet assures me it is time.

The veterinarian has me place a blanket and towels on the floor. First, she gives my girl a medication to make her drowsy and want to lie down. I hold her head. I am crying.

"It is okay to let go," I tell Hilton.

Her whole body becomes limp, and I know she is gone.

I weep.

The vet offers to give me a few minutes alone with her. I take some scissors and take a few cuttings of fur. Then the vet and her assistant take her to the car, wrapped in the blanket.

"The crematorium will pick up her body and return the ashes in a few weeks," the veterinarian informs me.

I chose a 'picture frame' urn for her with her paw print. A few weeks later, I receive it. I love it. I have a wonderful photo of her. I zoom in and crop, then have it printed nice and big. I will keep the ashes there until I find a place where I want to spread them.

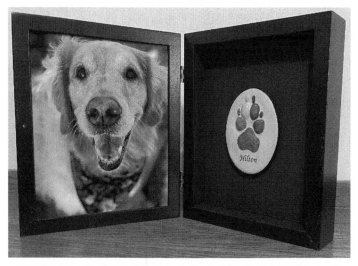

Just before Hilton's passing, I apply for another job at a chronic pain clinic and receive an interview. December 8th, 2021, one day after Hilton passes, I receive an offer for employment. When I'd interviewed for the position, I wasn't sure if I would accept it while Hilton was ill, as I would be away from home for much longer periods. I feel that Hilton passing is her way of saying I should take the job.

January 2022

After Hilton passes, things are tough, but I am determined to hold it together and not get depressed. I find a neighbourhood dog who would benefit from some walking (and training). So, I start to walk him almost daily. But the anxiety is getting more and more severe. Friends convince me I need to do something about it, and I find a therapist to talk to. I want to deal with my past traumas and be done. I am worried about being in therapy for the rest of my life.

I see the therapist, Tori, and start my new job. Anxiety subsides somewhat, but hunger becomes an issue. It becomes an intense hunger that never goes away. I can be starving or stuffed. It doesn't matter, as it was always there. I watch what I eat, but the sugar cravings are unbearable. I can't not eat it. We talk about how best to approach working on my previous trauma and begin to make plans when my life calms down a bit.

In March, I am working super long hours, both full time at my new job and part time at my old job. I am averaging fifty to sixty hours per week, and my mood starts to shift. I become hypomanic again. It starts mid-week, and by my Saturday morning appointment with Tori, I am very hypomanic. I'm talking fast, bouncing around physically and I suspect in my speech. Easily distracted, my senses are on high alert. I went off all antipsychotics during COVID, and I am determined not to go back on them.

When I am hypomanic, my symptoms usually consist of pressured and fast speech, the need to move my body, pursuing several interests at once, and my senses are extra perceptive: colours are brighter, sounds are louder, smells cause me bigger headaches and I can taste the smell. Any tight clothing feels uncomfortable, and I will wear oversized pants to cope. When I walk into Tori's office, I can immediately smell something perfumy. It takes us a few visits to figure out what the smell is—a small scented candle, never lit, that is on the opposite side of the room. It smells very strong to me, as though someone has spritzed the room with perfume.

When in this heightened state, I may alternate from not eating much to eating a bunch of junk. I try to force myself to go to bed and may or may not sleep well at night. I can become hyper-sexual, or spend a lot of money, both of which I may or may not regret later. Thankfully, this time, I avoid the hypersexuality and spending, but I do find myself more distracted on the right side.

It is difficult to explain what I mean by distracted more on my right side. It's kind of a visual distraction. I am aware of everything on my left, but I am much more aware of everything on my right. The colours are brighter. I notice more details, my attention is drawn to that side. But also, I notice how my clothing feels on the right side. I can feel the weight of my cochlear implant processor on my ear more on the right side.

I know it's time to worry during these episodes when I stop eating or sleeping reliably or when I develop delusions or hallucinations. My voices are all but gone; they are like a radio on in the background in another room. I am aware that they are there, but I can't hear what they are saying. I am trying not to give them any attention, as drawing attention to them makes them more powerful. I watch myself for sexual risk taking and spending lots of money. I know that becoming unable to drive or unable to focus at work are other signs to watch for that indicate it's time to contact my psychiatrist.

It's been about two-and-a-half weeks of this episode, and I continue to work. I actually work very well, as there are rules about having to work during work hours, and that keeps me on task. I am the kind of worker who is dedicated during the work hours. I have more difficulty in the off hours, doing home care work, as this is less structured, and it is easier to become distracted. For this reason, I decline home care referrals for a few weeks until I am feeling better. My strategy for working with clients is to take a breath before seeing them and purposefully slow myself down. I make a point to talk very little and allow the client to tell me what I need to know.

This specific episode starts to wane, and the auditory hangover returns. I am exhausted and I try to push myself to keep to my normal routine. Tori has to remind me that my body has been go-go-go for more than three weeks and it needs to rest. This helps me give myself permission to rest instead of trying to do anything and everything.

My sister has three kids, including a new baby. She stays with me when she comes to visit so my Gran can meet the baby. During this visit, I really start to realize how disconnected I am been from what 'normal' people feel. For example, one evening we are in the living room and the baby is in her crib in the bedroom. She starts to fuss and immediately my sister gets up to attend to her. I'm not saying I wouldn't do that if I had a kid as well, but it surprises me. Like *people actually get up and take care of their kids when they are upset?* It just kind of surprises me, since so much of my childhood happened without any kind of memorable affection from family in my household.

I talk to her a bit about my experience when I was at our childhood home and some of the things that I experienced. I am surprised by her reaction to how I was treated. I don't really understand how bad the situation at home sounds to someone like my sister, who wasn't there. To me, it just feels normal for my father to abandon me or his wife to try to get me out of the house. I am still shocked when my friends talk about their families being supportive of each other when growing up.

Late Spring 2022

Arguably, one could say I have been in hypomania for months now, even before my sister came to visit, and therefore, this episode is mania. However, I prefer to think of the previous months as me being well and happy. I don't like to think of the current episode as mania, although it probably is. Despite the length of time it has been ongoing, and the severity to which it is getting, I have been able to work and drive (with difficulty), and I have been able to continue to care for myself. I have been able to cope without changing my medications or ending up in a hospital. I can feel myself coming down. I am no longer vibrating with energy, talking a mile a minute, or tripping over my own thoughts. My senses have calmed, and the world is almost back to its normal self. The bright, vibrant, noisy, smelly, distracting world has calmed. I continue to have the agitation, which mostly is expressed as bouncing my legs, rubbing my pants, or rocking. Somehow, these movements seem to regulate my system and are an outlet for my agitation to be expressed.

At work, I mostly stick to myself during this time. I bounce my legs or swivel in my office chair, but I do not allow myself to show other signs of distress. I use all of my energy to stay still and calm with a client and make use of mindfulness techniques such as deep breathing and body scanning to slow myself down. When writing notes, I remove my processors if I need to reduce the distraction and stimulation that comes with the noises of the world.

Chapter 19

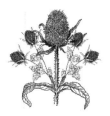

J UNE 2022

Sleep is not going well. I am averaging about four hours of sleep a night, yet I feel okay. My neighbour is selling his house, and there is no way I'm going to let their cheap, last-minute touch-ups make their house look better than mine. Unfortunately, while power washing the house, I decide it's a good idea to clean out the deck box and power wash it as well. The deck box is where I have been storing some of my garden supplies, mostly bags of soil and a few bags of rocks. Ignoring my own education and knowledge about body mechanics, I stupidly decide to lift a bag of rocks while leaning over the side of the deck box. While doing this, I pull my low back muscles and practically incapacitate myself.

This leads into a downward spiral. A neighbour gives me a Robax Platinum caplet with an Advil. I know that I'm not supposed to take NSAIDs with lithium, but I don't think one pill will make much of a difference. With the hospital having given me the shot of NSAID when I had the blood clot, I don't think a few pills will cause a problem. So, I take the pills and they help so much that I decide a few more days at a low dose couldn't possibly hurt. So, at the drugstore, I pick up some Acetaminophen-based Robaxacet and some Aleve, as it is only one pill every twelve hours. I take four pills over two days and notice that my tremor becomes worse. My first warning signal. However, I think nothing of it, as my tremor regularly varies in strength.

The week seems to go by fine from my perspective. I am busy as always. On Friday, I realize that my decision-making process might not be 100%, and I ask my CMHA caseworker, Olivia, if she might have time to go grocery shopping with me. I am worried that I will not make good decisions in the store and that I will come home with hundreds of dollars-worth of cookies (a half-exaggeration). Unfortunately, as it is last minute, she cannot help, as she is currently helping another client. I understand, especially since it is not like my cupboards are bare and I have a freezer with food. My problem is I need to menu plan ahead.

I decide, keeping with my decision to out-do my neighbour, that I will sand and stain the front veranda, protecting all the work I have done power washing the wood. I do not own a sander, and after a quick consideration and check online, I decide to purchase a battery-operated sander from the same line as my other power tools. It's even on sale and in stock locally! I purchase it with sandpaper, a sanding block, stain/protector, brushes, etc. When I get home and start sanding, I realize the batteries I own are only one-and-a-half amp and last about thirty minutes, which is barely enough time to make a dent in my sanding. Unable to feel frustration or concern about the cost, I go to another local hardware store that has a dual pack of the large batteries on sale and in stock. Altogether, I spent around $700 on tools and stains without batting an eye. This is my second warning signal, but I do not recognize it.

I spend nine hours on Saturday between the sanding and going to the store. My back is ready to give out, but I take only a few brief breaks. I worry I am annoying my neighbours with the constant whir of the sander, but I hope the final product will pay off for them. I cannot stain on Sunday, as it is going to rain, and even a bit of rain within twelve hours of application will ruin the finish. My house has become a disaster zone, so I use Sunday to clean it up. Dishes and stuff are everywhere. The sink has little white bits that are probably rice, but just might be maggots. I'm really not sure. However, I clean it up and run the dishwasher, determined to get my place in a slightly more acceptable state.

On Monday morning, the radio stations (except the local one) are all fuzzy, and my paranoia kicks in. My mind is worried. Black holes in the sky might be sucking up the radio waves. I know intellectually this can't be true, yet I still look. I calm myself a bit by asking a colleague if she noticed the radio being funny this morning; she did, and this calms me somewhat to know it was not just me who this is happening to.

Tuesday morning, I am up early and have been dancing since 6:30 a.m. with the music loud on the TV. As my neighbours are not home, I am taking advantage of the ability to blast music out loud. My anxiety is also non-existent, but I still do not recognize the warning signs of what is brewing around the corner.

Olivia stops by around 8:30 a.m. Tuesday. I had hoped to stain the full veranda on Monday evening. But because of a pop-up storm, it forced me to cover the railings with tarps and wait it out until Tuesday.

After our visit, I head to a nearby city for my home visit. On the way there, I realize things might not be quite right. My brain seems a bit fried, distracted, and when I visit, it takes all of my concentration to slow down and keep my speech making sense. By the time I am done and returning to work, I know I must take some time off. My team leader had already texted me that my afternoon appointment had been cancelled, and I ask her to cancel the rest of my week. I will come back to the office to finish up my leftover notes, then take a few days off to slow down.

I'm sure as soon as I get to the office, my team leader notices I am not right, but there is really nothing she can do. She cancels my appointments for this week. I need to sit down with one of the Nurse Practitioners to write a work letter for a patient before the Nurse Practitioner goes on holiday tomorrow. I can see on her face when she notices something is not right, and I can hear my speech is fast, pressured, and disorganized. She has that wide-eye, deer caught in a headlight look. "Can you order me a lithium level test?" I ask, trying to keep my speech clear and coherent. She agrees, as I am worried my lithium level is toxic. Later, in retrospect, I will realize it was probably toxic days ago, and what I am currently experiencing is residual effects from the off balance in my meds.

Wednesday, June 15th, 2022

Today, things are getting worse. I am off work, working around the house, and I can't stop. First, I am power washing the back deck, then I am pulling weeds; there are constantly things to do. I cannot drive myself to my appointment with Tori tonight, and after much debate, I ask my aunt, "Will you come stay the night with me?"

"What's the matter?" she asks.

"It's my mood. I'm manic. I can't drive tonight."

"Oh no. I'll come this afternoon," she says, with concern in her voice

She drops by in the afternoon, and she can discern I am unwell. I am constantly moving around, keeping busy. On Sunday, I made some tomato sauce base from my garden tomatoes. She fabulously turns it into delicious tomato soup and pasta sauce. I'm pretty impressed that my sauce turns out as well as it does, especially since I slightly burned it on Sunday when I forgot about it on the stove.

Anne takes me to my appointment with Tori, but my mind is running so quickly, I stutter when I speak.

"You need to message Olivia to see you asap tomorrow, as we can't do any work while you're manic," Tori directs me.

I think she has told me this once before, but honestly, all I can think about is Wednesday + 7:00 p.m. = appointment. My brain cannot process whether I should even go to this appointment or that I should be messaging Olivia.

I take some Ativan at night, which helps me get to fall asleep. However, I am awake again at 4:00 a.m. I sit in the warmth out on the front porch in the dark. Anne goes out later in the morning for some groceries when Olivia is supposed to arrive. I imagine to give me a little privacy. Olivia comes, and she, also, can tell I am not doing well. Although I am a little better than last night, I recognize intellectually that I should probably go to the hospital. I am stubborn and do not want to go. I am terrified of the hospital.

Eventually, I decide I should go. I realize I am likely to end up in the hospital if this keeps up, and at least this way it is on my terms, and I am empowered to choose when and where I go. Olivia drives me to the large psychiatric hospital in a city one hour away where the regional psychiatric hospital is located. I pack a bag and she cancels her afternoon appointments.

St Joe's main campus where the ER is located is an hour's drive, and I seem to calm and slow down a bit during the drive. We stop at Tim Hortons, since the ER will probably be a long wait. Once there, my anxiety increases, and I pace around the ER. I cannot stop, and my anxiety accelerates throughout the day. At one point I witness a lady getting handcuffed and brought into the psych ER, at which point I decide this is no longer a good idea and we need to leave. I beg Olivia, "Please, let's go."

She asks me, "why, what happened?" then insists, "You need to get looked at by a nurse."

I leave the ER completely and wait in the ambulance bay, begging her to leave through text. She won't go. I am frustrated, I am upset, I am desperate. She insists on waiting for the nurse, even though I need to get out of here.

Eventually, they call us into the psych ER, and it's exactly as I fear. It is behind a locked door, and I am treated inhumanely. First, I am scanned with a metal detector, then scanned with a wand, like some kind of criminal. They assigned me a dark cavernous room where one of two lights do not work and there is no furniture other than a hospital-style lazy boy chair. The entire room looks like an interview room, straight out of a TV police show. I do not want to enter. I am afraid that they will lock me in and never let me out.

The lady I saw previously being handcuffed and escorted into the psychiatric ER is constantly screaming, and they frequently call Code White for her. Every time I hear it, I am triggered back to my younger days when they would restrain me.

We wait for what seems like hours. I push to leave, but they won't let me until evaluated by a doctor. Eventually, another ER doctor comes.

"I won't be able to adjust your psych meds, as I'm not a psychiatrist."

"Well then, what good are you?" I don't mean it to be rude, but what was the point of wasting his time to come see me? A medical doctor has already seen me in the ER, who spoke to Olivia for all of two minutes before declaring that he would refer me to psychiatry.

I continue to pace in the hallway. Thankfully, they do not restrict me to the room. However, I am getting frustrated, as I am still waiting to be seen and I am hungry. The clerk finds me a sandwich and some snacks, and eventually a psychiatrist comes to the room.

We talk for a while, all while I am pacing the room. I am trying to explain to her what is going on, but I know that my thoughts are disjointed and rushed.

"My thoughts are like the keys in Harry Potter. If every thought were a key, when I try to grasp one, they all start flying a million miles a minute. Even when I do grasp one, if it is the right one, I have to use it quickly before it slips out of my hands."

She prescribes me something to slow me down, but when it comes, she has prescribed Olanzapine (Zyprexa), which I refuse to take. The nurse rolls her eyes, as if I am a bother because I know about psychiatric medications and what does or does not have negative side effects for me. The psychiatrist returns and, after further discussion, we agree on Ativan and Abilify to slow me down.

Once they have admitted me, Olivia brings in my bag and gets going. It's about 8:00 p.m. at this point. It has been a long day for both of us. I am taken via cab with a nurse to the West 5th campus (the Regional Psychiatric Hospital), where I am put on an acute floor. The floor sign still says 'concurrent disorders' but it is not, it is an acute floor now. The staff assess me throughout my stay. They like to ask about any hallucinations.

"Are you seeing or hearing anything that other people do not see or hear?"

My response is always the same—"Nothing different from usual."

They mistakenly take this as a 'no', which it is not. I've had the TV or radio on in the background in my head since 2016. That hasn't changed. I don't tell them 'yes' or 'no' because a) I don't want to lie b) I also don't want any extra antipsychotic medications c) I do not want to discuss the radio. If I leave them be, they do not bother me as much.

Friday, June 17th, 2022

The next day I realize what I have done (had myself admitted). I do not want to be in the hospital anymore and I am determined to get out. I will find a way even if I have to break into the key-card pads that secure the doors. My euphoric mania is changing, and I am now furious about being here. I pace the halls angrily and stutter as I speak. I yell, I slam doors; I make it known that I am not happy to be there. I am also angry about being bored. There is literally nothing for me to do, yet they won't let me have my laptop cord, which would keep me occupied and remedy much of the problem. They say it is a risk for me to have a cord, even sitting outside of the nursing station. Yet me being angry around the unit is not a risk... it makes little sense to me! The staff's solution to my boredom is medication. I sleep or colour with crayons. Neither of which is dignifying or a suitable solution to my problem.

During one of my rampages to get out, the doctor puts me on a Form. Until this point, they have considered me a voluntary patient, but with the Form he can keep me for fourteen days against my will. I am understandably pissed and even more determined to get out. I pack my bag angrily with my belongings and head to the doors. I pull the casings off the key swipes and attempt to figure out how to bypass the system.

"I am getting out of here." my speech is jumbled, and I stutter.

My thoughts fly all over. I don't get far between my distress and staff stopping me from breaking things. I sit on the floor to plot another method to escape.

There are a bunch of staff around me, but only one makes the effort to get down to my level, make eye contact with me, and talk to me directly. She is the social worker for the unit, and for the first time since getting there; I feel like someone is actually trying to help me. I continue to talk about the Harry Potter keys and black holes, but my mind is so jumbled I can't make sense of my speech, which is still presenting with a significant stutter.

They want to give me Seroquel, which I refuse. I eventually accept 2mg of Ativan from the staff as they get me back to my room and into bed. Later in the night, I become agitated again, and they give another

2mg of Ativan and get me settled again. I still have a bit of battery on my computer and write a brief note to myself. I cannot concentrate enough to spell.

Journal Entry – Friday June 17, 2022
I have only been here a few days and taken the Abilify twice. They keep offering me Haloperidol and Olanzapine, which I refuse to take. But even just those 2 doses of Abilify and already I can't focus. I am having difficulty typign these sentenses as I try to wrtie this. I obciouslys cannot stay on this medicaion long. I won't be able to work. I am trying to keep my normal schedule: wake around 545, bed around 1115. But they keep forcing medicaions on me when I get agitated during the day. Can you blame me? They got me locked up in a little unit with 2 hallways to walk around. No wonder I'm going stir crazy. But no, they don't care. As far as they are concerned I am on a form and just have to deal with it I I no longer have a say in anything..

It has taken 4mg of Ativan to slow me down enough for my thoughts to be linear, yet I still cannot spell correctly.

Saturday, June 18th, 2022

Today I am once again aggravated, bored, and frustrated. I want out. A nurse offers me a choice of four books, none of which I am interested in, and even if I was, I cannot concentrate. So, I reject them. She offers me pills, but already feeling hungover, I decline. Most of the day I am tired because of the medications, but when they wear off, I am in that in-between zone where I am not quite sedated and getting angry. As a result, I bang on objects around the unit. Doors, sanitizer dispensers, etc. while pacing the halls. Not hard, just enough to make a noise.

Suddenly, there are security personnel. They have not given me any opportunity to be helped to calm down. Just poof—they show up.

"You are going to seclusion or security will go hands on," the nurse tells me

Naturally, I do what any person would do—I turn away. I head for my room. They take my desire for privacy to discuss the matter as a sign of resistance. But I'm not resisting (although I certainly do not want to go), I just want privacy to discuss and instead I am suddenly assaulted and held to the ground by security as I fight for my life. Staff have unnecessarily escalated the situation without giving me a chance or even proper warning. They have not offered me any more medication nor said, "You need to take this or you will end up in seclusion." I have not been told to go to my room to calm down, or encouraged to seek support from friends or family. I receive no warning that I will soon be removed from the unit if I don't calm down.

So, I fight back, of course I fight back.

"You're going into seclusion," they tell me as I am being assaulted.

They pin me to the ground.

"You can either calm down enough and walk with us or we will restrain you to a wheelchair," Nurse Ratched informs me.

In absolute fear of restraint, I shut myself down enough to walk with them, all while being held forcefully. They hold me so forcefully my arms bruise.

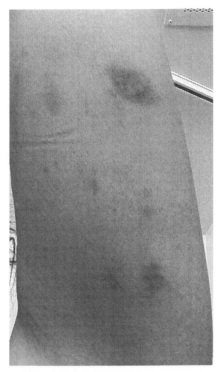

In the seclusion room, which is upstairs, there is a mattress on the floor, two cups of water, a bedpan, and two cardboard urinals. I am forced to lie face down on the mattress with the full weight of security on me. I feel like a felon. They kneel on me so hard I worry they will cut off my ability to breathe. I am terrified that they will sedate me, and so I scream over and over that I do not consent. After a few minutes, despite them talking to me without being able to see their faces, I understand they will let me go as long as I don't move while they leave the room. They check my sweater for strings and my pockets for my phone (which has fallen out onto the floor in my room). Then they take my shoes and leave me.

Being in seclusion is terrible for anyone. It is a small room, about eight by ten feet in size. There is only a small window facing the hall, just big enough for the staff to check on the trapped patient. They dim the lights, restricting my vision, in addition to my current hearing loss and the lack of sound in the room. It is so isolating.

At first I fight it, determined to find a way out. The nurse comes back after a few minutes with security (as if I am some kind of danger to others) and gives me some pills to calm me; 2mg of Ativan in addition to my normal medications. I know I am stuck here for the night and fighting will do no good. I resign myself and lay on the mattress, broken and numb. To get through this, I tell myself to just play dead.

Being in seclusion is terrible for anyone. The staff justifies putting me in seclusion by saying I am overstimulated and need to 'de-stim'. So, they take me from being in an overstimulated environment to an under-stimulated one. One torture to another. I am left in this room with nothing to do, nothing to look at, nothing to listen for except the noises in my head. It deprives my senses. I calm down, but not because I am de-stimulated, as they think, but because I have given up. I succumb to my fate and retreat into my mind. They've broken my spirit and called it successful treatment.

· In the middle of the night, I have to go to the bathroom, but they will not let me out. I decide to tear a cardboard urinal and create a bigger hole and use it over the bedpan, hoping that it will reduce the urine smell overnight. My sense of smell is so sensitive that I cannot imagine enduring that smell all night. I seem to do an okay job and I don't think I spill much, and whatever misses lands in the bedpan. However, the entire process is degrading and I feel inhuman.

In the morning, a new nurse brings me a breakfast tray and places it on the floor. There is no table or chairs, therefore I must eat seated on the floor like a dog, completely dehumanized. I resign and sit with my legs straight out and my back leaning against the wall to try to down some cold oatmeal with a plastic spoon.

"We will try a trial-out in a few hours," the nurse says, "To see if you are ready to go back to the unit."

A 'trial-out' is basically a test run. They let you out, but with the constant overhang that they have the power to throw you back in at any little indiscretion. Another threat, this one unspoken. I am calm. Why can't I go back now? I wonder, but I know better than to say anything that could be perceived the wrong way and risk being left in this hole any longer.

The new nurse comes to retrieve me from the seclusion room a few hours later and allows me to use the bathroom, which turns out to be right next door. Before she frees me, she makes me repeat, like a toddler in time out, why they put me in seclusion. I am broken; I don't care. I will do whatever I can to be let out of this room; so, I tell her what she wants to hear.

"I was banging walls and out of control."

She does not know how much this experience has set me back in my healing. All this because of a few bangs on the wall.

Over the next few days, the medications filter out of my system. My fatigue dissipates and my concentration returns. I talk to the doctor about leaving, but the staff encourages me to stay and get the meds sorted out. I do not want to take the Abilify, and so I refuse that, and he agrees to take down the Epival to 350 mg once daily to reduce the somnolence and hunger. He also agrees to add the Wellbutrin, which I know historically has always returned my depression to a more neutral level.

While on the unit, the social worker assists me to fill out paperwork for Employment Insurance. My manager has offered to send in the appropriate forms for sick leave. This will provide me with a small income for the time that I am off work, which will be beneficial. I also receive an email from the ADP program, which is the program which funds mobility devices for people in Ontario. They are requesting information on clients I saw between 2018 and 2021. I return their email explaining that I am in the hospital and therefore cannot provide what they want at the moment. They respond in a few days with an extension. This time I ask the social worker to email them and let them know I cannot provide this information at present and cannot provide an estimate of when I will be able to do so.

I spend four weeks in the unit, getting my health sorted out. My aunt brings me toiletries that I have forgotten and comes to visit me one day. I get passes to leave the unit, to go down to Tim Hortons. At first, I am worried that I will see someone I know. Eventually, I stop caring. The hospital is new, opened in 2014, and has an advanced security system. Everything is on access cards, and the entrance to the inpatient units has a security check. This creates two areas with varying levels of passes, allowing patients to leave the unit but not be able to go beyond security.

On the inpatient side of security there is a small cafe, a gym, and a games room. Most of the inpatient units have a small exercise room that patients can get cleared to use. Outside of security, there is a Tim Hortons and cafeteria. There are also services, including x-ray, MRI, and various mental and non-mental health outpatient clinics.

While I am hospitalized, I let a few people know I am once again in the hospital. I have little understanding of consequences, so while I would usually never speak of my mental health to anyone, I tell several friends. To my surprise, one night my friend Lawrence shows up, excited to see me. I am surprised and delighted to have a visitor, even if I am just getting ready for bed. I do not have passes to leave the campus, so we sit downstairs in the empty cafeteria. Everything is closed, but it doesn't matter. We catch up for an hour. Lawrence is Deaf and we use ASL. It is so nice to not struggle to communicate. Nurses on the unit wear masks, and between the background noise, yelling from other patients, and my current mental status, listening is hard, tiring, and something I am struggling to do.

It is nice to see him, and we hug on his way out. I see him a week later when we go out for lunch to a place he used to go to as a kid down by the water. Another day, he picks me up and drives to his old childhood home. He shows me where he grew up, which is close to the McDonald's we are going to for food. He visits me three times, and I am thankful for him as a friend.

My psychiatrist at the hospital has to be the coolest psychiatrist I have ever met. He is an older black man with dreads and with just a touch of grey. He dresses well and one day he wears a dark-pink checkered suit. He is laid back and genuine. I am awake and alert as he makes his rounds each morning at 7:45am. We often chat for 10-15 minutes. I really feel like he listens to me and considers my input. He tries me on various drugs, including Epival, Ativan, Clonazepam, Wellbutrin SR, and Abilify. I refuse the Abilify after a few days, and the Clonazepam makes me combative.

I am always restless in hospitals, and this time is no different. I walk the halls all day and sometimes all night. One day I walk 57,591 steps or 42.71 kilometres just by pacing the unit. My ankle becomes so sore that I cannot bear weight on it. The doctor approves me to use crutches and I get an x-ray to confirm I do not have a stress fracture. As a result of this pacing, I am not too concerned about my increase in hunger. I am aware of it and am careful to limit the servings I eat. Sadly, it does not work, and when I come home, I will be ten pounds heavier than I was just four weeks previously.

They allow me to go home for two weekends to prepare for discharge. The first weekend, I plan to drive my car back to the hospital so that I can drive myself home later next week when discharged. Unfortunately, I realize I am not ready to face city driving. I struggle to drive just ten minutes on empty country roads; accordingly, I ask my aunt or uncle to drive me back to the hospital on Sunday.

It seems like it is time for discharge next week. I return from the weekend pass with a stuffed-up head from allergies, as the hospital has not been giving me my allergy medication. I spend a few low-key days in my room, as I'm feeling poorly being congested. This low-key behaviour indicates to the doctor I am ready to be discharged and discharge begins.

"You can go home on Thursday," the doctor says.

My aunt and uncle, who have been doing the driving up to this point, are away, so one of my best friends, Megan, plans to take me home.

July 14th, 2022

As luck would have it, the week when I am to come home, both Tori and Olivia are on vacation. Olivia has arranged for me to be helped by one of her colleagues, who I have texted to let her know I will go home today. Even though we conversed ahead of time, that she would wear a mask (if required), and being discreet (as I don't want neighbours to see a medical person entering my home), she presumed we were going to check in via text. This also makes no sense because Olivia had asked her to help me check that I have food and to go grocery shopping if needed. Anyway, Megan has time to help, and we clean out the fridge and go shopping. However, she is the first to admit that she is not a mental health worker and is not really sure how to support me in that regard.

Once I leave the hospital, I quickly figure out that I am always hungry and always seething with anger in the morning. I remember that I have taken the Epival before but can't remember why I stopped it. I ask my community psychiatrist when I get out of the hospital.

"You had stopped it previously because of the weight gain," he says to me.

A few days later, I realize the anger is coming from the low amount of Wellbutrin in my system first thing in the morning. Therefore, shortly after taking the Wellbutrin SR, my anger subsides. I ask for an urgent appointment over the phone with my psychiatrist, so later that week I have a longer call with him. I want off the Epival and switched to the Wellbutrin XL (I have already begun taking my old pills with improvement in my mood). My psychiatrist reminds me I am not one of those people who can go off medication, and I agree, but I am not willing to take a medication that makes me starving 24/7 and is responsible in part for me gaining so much weight (the Epival) nor take a medication that makes me so angry every morning (the Wellbutrin SR). He finally agrees.

"Okay. You can cut your dose of the Epival in half each week for two weeks," he says.

He puts me on half my previous dose of the Wellbutrin XL (now 150mg), even though I felt good these past few days on the 300mg.

The hunger is persisting, although lessening with the smaller dose of Epival. I am trying to limit my calories, but the hunger is so persistent, it's nearly impossible. I am hungry, so I eat. If I do not eat, I am hangry. If I get hangry, I still eat, but I eat junk. I lose either way. At the end of July, I weigh 195 pounds. I feel bloated, fat, and disgusting, and barely any of my clothing fits.

Conclusion

F ALL 2022

I am feeling much better now, and my medications are more stable. My regimen includes an antihistamine and propranolol every morning, and lithium, Vraylar, and Wellbutrin XL at night. Strangely, I do better with the Wellbutrin XL at night. It is supposed to be a more activating medication, and for that reason, most people take it in the morning. I have also started an injectable medication called Ozempic to help with hunger. After getting over the initial fear of giving myself a needle, it has reduced my hunger to a more reasonable level. I am still increasing the dose, but we do this slowly so my body can accommodate.

Work is going well. I feel I am back to myself, minus some social anxiety, and able to help patients to the best of my ability. I had no problems returning gradually to work. My fears of being fired because of my mental health were unfounded. I am currently co-teaching a group about pain, developing a group about returning to work, and connecting with a local seniors' centre for providing pain-related programming to their members.

I still hear 'voices'; it's really more like a radio or tv in the background. Sometimes it's a laugh track, other times it's run on speech, like a newscaster. In any case, I usually cannot tell what they are saying. It usually comes from behind me, to the left. I try not to talk about it much. I find when I talk about it, it gives it power. It makes it more prominent in my head. So, instead, I respond to questions vaguely. In the hospital they asked if I was hearing anything, to which I would respond "nothing different from usual". This is my way of saying yes—I hear something, but it's not a concern, I can deal with it. I don't want medication for this.

My fear of the hospital has lessened somewhat, and I can now recognize that it can help when things are terrible. That being said, I am still terrified of seclusion or restraints, and it will be difficult for me in the future to go to the hospital as long as I know those are a possibility. I am working with Tori to make a binder regarding how to help me if/when I become sick again. Things that I know help but might not be able to tell the hospital staff in that situation.

My relationship with my grandmother is still strong, and my ability to open up to my mom's family is increasing. I still do not talk to my father, nor do I have any desire to.

I still struggle with the damage inflicted by the medical staff in the mental health programs and hospitals while I was in high school. The ones who told me, time after time, that I was the problem. That I was making it up. That I wanted attention. Those small brief moments of blame did nothing to help me heal and only made me worse. I have to work to not allow myself to take the blame for everything that goes wrong or to accept other people's problems as my responsibility. I am working on not being mistreated and taken advantage of by people I care about that may be having a bad day. I learn I am not the reason all is not right in the world.

I am thankful for the various medical staff who made a difference by really caring. My doctor at McMaster did not have to take five minutes out of her busy day to walk me to the ambulance. But she did, and that made me feel like someone cared and things would be okay. In Toronto, a hospital ombudsman listened to me despite my obviously unwell state and then made sure I made it back to the ER, with Hilton, for the help that I needed.

I am thankful for my various CMHA caseworkers who made sure I got to my medical appointments when I was unable to do so independently. There is the Early Psychosis Intervention nurse, who technically did not work for CMHA (but I saw her in their building), who patiently waited for me to work up the courage to allow her to give me my injected medications for several years. Olivia, who spent twelve hours with me and sat all day in the ER to make sure I got the help I needed. There was the social worker this most recent time in the hospital, who got down on my level and made eye contact, really trying to get through to me despite my floridly manic state. I thank Tori, who has listened to my anxiety since January and helped me work through a lot of my issues surrounding hospitalization and with allowing and trusting people to know what is going on in my life. With her encouragement, I have written this book, and maybe someday I'll even share it with friends, family, and the public.

If I could say one thing to all the medical staff and mental health workers out there, it would be to *be the person who cares. Be the person who makes a difference.* You never know what little act may help a patient feel like someone cares and that can change the course of an episode.

Finally, I want to thank all of my friends, family, and co-workers who have put up with my nuttiness, my anxiety, and my mood swings for all of these years. I would not have made it this far without you.

Dear Reader:
Did you enjoy reading RESILIENT?
Please consider writing a review on Amazon.
Reviews help non-traditionally published books get
exposure, reach a wider audience and make a greater
impact.